Olena Berezovska

Growing Up Strong:

A Guide to Girls' Health and Well-Being

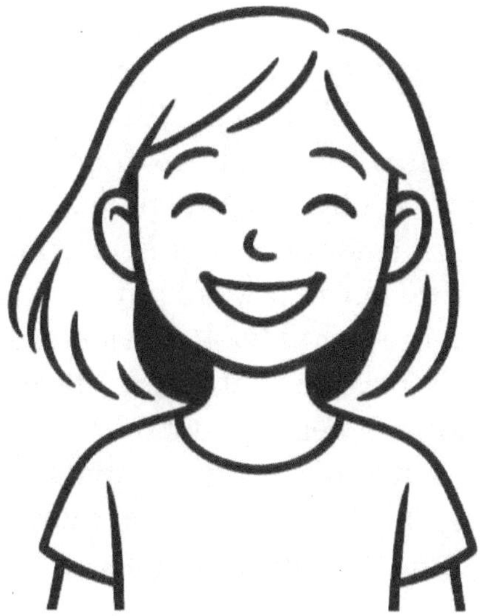

International Academy of Healthy Life

2025

Growing Up Strong: A Guide to Girls' Health and Well-Being

Olena Berezovska

Publisher: International Academy of Healthy Life

Description:

This comprehensive guide explores girls' unique health and developmental needs from birth to adulthood. Growing Up Strong is an invaluable resource for parents, caregivers, and educators, covering everything from physical growth, hormonal changes, and reproductive health to emotional well-being, mental health, and social influences. Written by renowned physician and author Olena Berezovska, this evidence-based book provides practical advice and insights on nurturing girls through every stage of their journey, empowering them to lead healthy, confident, and fulfilling lives. Whether addressing nutrition, puberty, mental health challenges, or societal pressures, this book offers the knowledge and tools to support girls in reaching their full potential.

This essential guide celebrates girls' resilience and strength, equipping readers with the understanding and confidence to help them thrive in a rapidly changing world.

Table of contents

From the Author

Dear Readers: Mothers, Fathers, and Young Girls,

This book is for anyone interested in understanding and supporting girls' health from birth through the completion of puberty. It provides a forward-looking perspective, envisioning a girl's journey toward becoming a woman, a wife, a mother, and perhaps one day, someone who will raise her children.

I have wanted to create a book specifically focused on girls' health for many years. This vital topic remains surprisingly underrepresented in both popular and medical literature.

As a woman, I have experienced growth, puberty, and the transition to adulthood, including motherhood. This gives me a uniquely "female" perspective — a lived experience no man can fully replicate or understand.

I also have a daughter who grew up entirely under my care, without reliance on external caregivers. Through close observation of her growth and development, I witnessed every stage of her transformation firsthand. Our warm and open relationship and my interactions with her friends gave me unique insights into the needs, concerns, fears, and misconceptions that often accompany a young girl's journey, particularly during adolescence.

As a doctor, I can combine my experiences with professional expertise in gynecology, the medical field dedicated to women's health. Over the years, I have worked closely with parents and their daughters, listened to their stories, and addressed their questions and concerns. My experience in health education, including delivering lectures on puberty and related topics in schools, has further deepened my understanding of the challenges young girls face. These lectures, often aimed at children and teenagers, have reinforced the importance of providing clear and accurate information.

One of the motivations for writing this book stems from the increasing commercialization of healthcare. Healthcare has become a commodity in some regions, where diagnoses and treatments are often driven by profit rather than genuine need. This trend has led to the overuse of diagnostic tests and many expensive, unnecessary, and aggressive treatments that are sometimes invasive and unjustified. Unfortunately, pediatric gynecology has not been immune to these practices. In many countries, there is a glaring lack of specialized training in girls' health, and existing resources are often outdated or inadequate. Yet, paradoxically, unwarranted medical interventions in young girls' lives are on the rise, starting from birth.

This book aims to address these gaps. It offers clear, evidence-based guidance for parents and young girls, empowering them to make informed and mindful decisions for a healthier future.

It's important to remember that a child's life is about much more than doctor visits, tests, and vaccinations, although these remain essential components of health. Raising a healthy child requires constant effort, care, and attention from parents. Health begins even before birth and is shaped by a woman's physical well-being during pregnancy and the environmental conditions in which a child is raised. Factors like nutrition, rest, activity, family relationships, and emotional well-being are critical to a child's health.

In 2018, my book *Дочки-матери: Все, о чем вам не рассказывала ваша мама и чему стоит научить свою дочь* (*Daughters and Mothers: Everything Your Mother Didn't Tell You and What You Should Teach Your Daughter*) was published in Russia and became a bestseller. Its success highlighted the urgent need for accessible, comprehensive, and accurate information on girls' health.

This English edition represents a significant step forward. It includes many new chapters and updated evidence-based information reflecting the latest scientific research and medical guidelines. Writing this edition in English is particularly important because it makes this crucial knowledge available to a broader, global audience, ensuring that more families can benefit from accurate and practical insights into raising healthy girls.

In this book, I delve into many aspects of girls' development, shedding light on often-overlooked issues in children's health. My goal is to equip you with knowledge and understanding to help you nurture a healthy, thriving girl, both physically and emotionally.

This book is a valuable resource for your family and inspires you on this critical journey.

Happy reading!

Olena Berezovska

How Does a Girl Begin?

What we do know is that a child's sex is determined by a complex interplay of factors, beginning with the **sex chromosomes**. Chromosomes are thread-like structures found in nearly every cell of the human body. They carry **DNA (deoxyribonucleic acid)**, a molecule that contains the instructions for building and maintaining a living organism. DNA is divided into **genes**, which control specific traits such as eye color, height, and how the body functions. Together, chromosomes serve as the blueprint for the human body, holding the key to understanding how life begins and unfolds.

Each human typically has **46 chromosomes** arranged in **23 pairs**. These include **22 pairs of autosomes**, which are chromosomes the same in both males and females. Autosomes carry most of the body's genetic instructions but play a minimal role in determining sex differences. The **23rd pair** consists of the sex chromosomes, directly determining biological sex. A complete set of chromosomes in a person is called a **karyotype**, and it can be visualized through a diagnostic process called **karyotyping**, which is often used to identify a child's sex or detect certain genetic disorders.

In women, the karyotype is **46 XX**, meaning they have two **X chromosomes**. These chromosomes are identical in structure but come from different origins – one from the mother and one from the father. In men, the karyotype is **46 XY**, meaning they inherit one **X chromosome** from their mother and one **Y chromosome** from their father. This difference in the X and Y chromosomes determines biological sex at the chromosomal level.

Sex determination begins at the moment of conception, when a single sperm cell fertilizes a female egg, forming a new, unique cell called a **zygote**. The zygote is a new human's first cell, containing 46 chromosomes – half from the mother and half from the father. The egg always contributes an X chromosome since women only have X chromosomes to pass on. However, sperm cells can carry either an X or Y chromosome. If a sperm carrying an X chromosome fertilizes the egg, the zygote will have an XX karyotype, and the child will be female. If a sperm carrying a Y chromosome fertilizes the egg, the zygote will have an XY karyotype, and the child will be male. Therefore, the child's sex is entirely determined by which sperm fertilizes the egg, making the father's genetic contribution decisive in this process.

While the mother does not directly influence the child's sex, her body plays a vital role in supporting the conception process. After sperm enters the female reproductive tract during intercourse, it embarks on a challenging journey. It must travel from the vagina, through the uterus, and into the fallopian tubes, where the egg is waiting. Along the way, the sperm encounters various natural selection mechanisms, such as the acidity of the vaginal environment and the structure of cervical mucus. These mechanisms can influence the survival and quality of the sperm, and some researchers speculate that they might subtly affect whether a boy (Y chromosome) or a girl (X chromosome) is conceived. However, this remains a topic of ongoing scientific investigation.

Despite the complexity of this process, the global ratio of boys to girls at birth has remained remarkably stable over centuries. On average, about **101 boys are born for every 100 girls**, resulting in a near **1:1 ratio**. This balance may vary slightly across populations due to environmental, genetic, or cultural factors. For instance, in some regions, societal preferences or medical interventions have shifted natural sex ratios. However, on a global scale, this equilibrium persists. Interestingly, the 1:1 ratio is unique to humans, as other species often have sex ratios that vary significantly depending on environmental pressures or reproductive strategies.

It's also worth noting that while sex determination is primarily a matter of chromosomes, other factors may shape reproductive patterns. For example, some studies suggest that environmental conditions such as stress or parental age could influence sex ratios in specific populations, though these effects are minor and not fully understood.

Ultimately, sex determination is a complex process guided by the intricate interplay of genetics, biology, and natural selection. The zygote's formation marks the beginning of a remarkable journey of growth, development, and identity, which we will explore in greater detail throughout this book.

Did You Know?

- *The father's sperm determines a baby's sex, as it carries either an X or a Y chromosome.*
- *Humans have a nearly 1:1 birth ratio of boys to girls, a balance unique among species.*

From Chromosomes to Gonads

Once a child is conceived, the sex chromosomes play a critical role in determining biological sex. In female and male embryos, the **gonads**, organs that eventually develop into **ovaries or testes**, begin forming. These organs are essential for the reproductive system, enabling the body to produce offspring as it matures. However, gonads serve two interconnected functions beyond reproduction:

1. **Production and Maturation of Sex Cells**: These **gametes**, eggs in females and sperm in males, carry half of the genetic material necessary for reproduction.
2. **Hormone Production**: Hormones act as chemical messengers that regulate reproduction, growth, and the development of secondary sexual characteristics, such as breast development in girls and voice deepening in boys.

While these functions start during embryonic development, they only fully activate after puberty, when the body can reproduce.

In the earliest stages of development, gonads in all embryos are **bipotential**, meaning they can develop into either ovaries or testes, regardless of the embryo's chromosomal composition (XX for females, XY for males). This stage, known as **bipotentiality**, lasts only a few days after conception. The process of **sexual**

differentiation, the development of male or female physical characteristics, soon begins, guided primarily by the sex chromosomes.

In embryos with a Y chromosome (XY), a specific gene located on this chromosome, the **SRY gene** (*Sex-determining Region Y*), acts as a master switch for male development. The SRY gene produces a protein known as the **testis-determining factor (TDF)**, which initiates a cascade of genetic events leading to the development of testes. Testes produce small amounts of testosterone, the hormone responsible for male-specific structures like the *vas deferens (a* tube that carries sperm) and *seminal vesicles* (glands that contribute to semen).

In embryos with two X chromosomes (XX), the absence of the SRY gene allows the gonads to develop into ovaries naturally. This process occurs slightly later than testicular development in XY embryos, reflecting what researchers call a "waiting period." Without the SRY-triggered signals, other genes activate to promote ovarian development while suppressing male-specific genes. Female development involves specific genetic and molecular pathways, including the roles of RSPO1 and WNT4, which promote ovarian formation and suppress male-specific traits. During this phase, the hormonal environment in female embryos remains relatively quiet, as ovaries do not produce significant amounts of hormones until later in fetal development.

This natural progression from bipotential gonads to sex-specific organs highlights the delicate interplay of genetic and hormonal signals determining whether an embryo develops as male or female. While female development has traditionally been viewed as the "default" pathway, modern research continues to uncover the intricate mechanisms that make both processes equally complex and fascinating.

Unlike male embryos, which rely on the active signaling of specific genes like SRY, no equivalent "female" genes have been identified that directly guide ovarian development. Instead, female development proceeds in the absence of male-specific signals. This absence highlights the critical role of male-determining genes, while female differentiation relies on the coordinated activation and suppression of various genetic pathways.

In both male and female embryos, **primary sex cells**, the precursors to eggs and sperm, originate outside the embryo in a structure called the **yolk sac**. From there, these cells migrate to the gonads (testes in males and ovaries in females). This migration is a vital step for proper reproductive development. For males, these cells eventually relocate externally to the scrotum, where the testes reside.

During their early development, these primary sex cells undergo **mitotic division**, increasing their numbers. At this stage, they remain bipotential, meaning they can develop into either male or female sex cells. Surprisingly, this process is not controlled by sex chromosomes or specific male or female genes but rather by poorly understood mechanisms.

In male embryos, the program for **spermatogenesis** (sperm development) begins around 12.5 days after conception (approximately the 4th obstetric week of pregnancy). While this early program sets the foundation for producing male sex cells, it remains dormant until puberty, when the testes become fully functional.

In female embryos, the program for **oogenesis** (egg development) activates one day later, on the 13th day after conception. At this point, the primary sex cells begin **meiotic division**, a specialized process that halves the chromosome number, preparing the cells for reproduction. Unlike in males, female embryos complete this initial division stage before birth. The eggs then enter a suspended, immature state until puberty triggers their final maturation and release during **ovulation**.

Male development is often considered "active," as it depends on activating specific genes like SRY and testosterone production. By contrast, female

development is described as "passive," occurring without male-specific signals. However, this characterization is misleading, as female development involves finely tuned genetic and hormonal processes as intricate as those driving male differentiation.

What Parents and Daughters Should Know About Ovarian Health

A fascinating aspect of female reproduction is that a woman's **ovarian reserve**, the total number of eggs she will ever have, is established before birth. This finite supply begins to decline naturally, even before puberty. By the time a girl reaches puberty, only a fraction of these eggs remains, and only a tiny number will mature and be released during ovulation.

Because the ovarian reserve is non-renewable, any damage to the ovaries or nearby **pelvic organs** (due to surgeries, injuries, or specific medical treatments) can significantly impact a woman's reproductive potential. Such disruptions may lead to a reduced ovarian reserve, early **menopause**, or even **infertility**. Parents can play a crucial role in educating their daughters about protecting their reproductive health. Simple practices such as avoiding unnecessary procedures and being mindful of environmental and lifestyle factors can help preserve fertility.

Teaching girls to value and care for their reproductive health empowers them to make informed decisions about their bodies, ensuring their well-being now and in the future.

Did You Know?

- *In early development, all embryos have gonads that can become either ovaries or testes, regardless of their sex chromosomes.*
- *A woman's total number of eggs is determined before birth and cannot be replenished, making ovarian health vital for lifelong fertility.*

From Gonads to Hormones

By now, you understand that a child's sex is determined by the sex chromosomes inherited from their parents, the formation of reproductive organs, primarily the gonads (ovaries and testes), and the appearance of primary sex cells within them. However, these essential factors alone are not enough. A girl won't fully develop as a girl, nor a boy as a boy, without the powerful influence of **sex hormones**.

There are two primary groups of sex hormones in the human body. **Male sex hormones**, collectively called **androgens**, include **testosterone**, which is responsible for male traits such as muscle growth, deepening of the voice, and the production of sperm. **Female sex hormones**, known as **estrogens**, include several forms, with **estradiol** being the most dominant and playing a key role in the development of female traits like breast growth, menstrual cycles, and maintaining bone health.

Sex hormones are part of a more prominent family of chemicals called **steroid hormones** derived from **cholesterol** (a type of fat found in the body). In addition to androgens and estrogens, this group includes **progesterone**, which is crucial for maintaining pregnancy; adrenal hormones like **cortisol**, which helps the body manage stress; and **aldosterone**, which regulates salt and water balance.

Although progesterone is not classified as a strict sex hormone, it plays a significant role in reproduction. For example, progesterone prepares the uterus for pregnancy, maintains the uterine environment to support the growing fetus, and helps prevent premature contractions.

The role of sex hormones has been extensively studied across various animal models, shedding light on their influence during development. For example, introducing androgens or estrogens into the embryos of many animals can override the influence of their chromosomes, triggering the growth of testes or ovaries, even in embryos with opposing chromosomal compositions. This demonstrates the immense power of these hormones in shaping reproductive organs and secondary sexual traits.

In humans, the chromosomal composition (XX or XY) provides the "blueprint" for development, but sex hormones act as the "builders," carrying out the instructions encoded in the chromosomes. Their presence, timing, and levels are critical for proper sexual development and differentiation.

In 1987, researchers proposed a theory suggesting that sexual differentiation depends on the **ratio** of sex hormones androgens (male hormones) to estrogens (female hormones) rather than their absolute levels. This balance determines whether the gonads develop into testes or ovaries and guides the broader differentiation of the fetus into a male or female.

Specific genes, such as **CYP19** (aromatase), regulate this balance. **Aromatase** is an enzyme that converts testosterone into estradiol, ensuring a proper hormonal environment for development. This process is critical during early pregnancy when any disruption to this balance can cause abnormalities in sexual differentiation.

Understanding the critical role of sex hormones in development highlights the potential dangers of external hormonal exposure during pregnancy. The unnecessary use of hormones, especially in high doses, during the early stages of fetal development can interfere with the natural processes of sex differentiation. This may lead to developmental defects, improper formation of reproductive organs, or complications in sexual development later in life.

For this reason, healthcare providers must exercise caution when prescribing hormonal treatments during pregnancy. Expectant mothers should also avoid self-medicating with hormone-related drugs or supplements, as even small exposures can have lasting impacts on a child's reproductive health.

Did You Know?

- *Sex hormones like testosterone and estradiol shape not only reproductive organs but also secondary traits like voice depth and bone health.*
- *Disruptions in the balance of sex hormones during pregnancy can affect a child's sexual development and reproductive health for life.*

From Hormones to Sexual Characteristics

The final stage of **sexual differentiation**, or **sex determination**, is the development of the **male or female phenotype**, the physical and internal traits that distinguish one sex from another. **Phenotype** refers to observable characteristics shaped by genetics, hormones, and environmental influences. These include physical features like skin tone, hair and eye color, body structure, facial attributes, and internal traits like the structure and function of reproductive organs.

While internal structures such as gonads and reproductive organs are vital to sexual function, external features like genitalia and secondary sexual characteristics, traits that appear during puberty, play a key role in defining male and female phenotypes. The interaction between chromosomes, gonads, and hormones drives these differences. A disruption at any level of this process can result in atypical sexual traits or reproductive challenges.

Sex hormones, such as testosterone and estrogens like estradiol, are central to the development of male and female characteristics. These hormones act as "messengers," translating genetic instructions into physical traits. For instance:

- **Testosterone** stimulates the development of male features such as muscle growth, facial hair, and deepening of the voice.

- **Estradiol**, the dominant estrogen in females, promotes breast development, fat distribution, and the regulation of menstrual cycles.

Sex hormones exert their effects independently of genes in some contexts. Administering testosterone or estrogen, for example, can induce male or female traits, regardless of chromosomal makeup. It is evident in clinical treatments, such as:

- Testosterone therapy for delayed puberty in boys.
- Estrogen therapy for managing menopausal symptoms or supporting feminization in transgender women.

Additionally, research on **reversible sex determination** in animal models shows that altering hormone levels can override genetic signals, emphasizing the decisive role of hormonal balance.

However, the effects of sex hormones are dose-dependent and ratio-sensitive. A shift in the androgen-to-estrogen ratio can disrupt normal development, leading to conditions like ambiguous genitalia or delayed secondary sexual traits.

Genetic and hormonal signals influence the processes of **feminization** (development of female traits) and **masculinization** (development of male traits). Genes located on autosomal chromosomes (the 22 non-sex chromosomes shared by males and females) play a critical role in regulating reproduction and the development of internal organs. Mutations or defects in these genes can lead to infertility or atypical sexual development.

Externally, boys and girls differ primarily in **primary sexual characteristics** and genital structures at birth. However, during **puberty**, a surge in sex hormone production triggers the development of **secondary sexual characteristics**, which further define male and female phenotypes:

- **In males**, secondary traits include the growth of facial and body hair, increased muscle mass, and a deepened voice.
- **In females**, these traits include breast development, widening of the hips, and changes in fat distribution.

Internally, these processes shape the reproductive organs and their functions. For example:

- In males, the testes produce sperm and testosterone.

- In females, the ovaries produce eggs, estrogen, and progesterone.

Sexual differentiation is not a single event but an ongoing process that begins during fetal development and extends into adulthood. During fetal life, the groundwork is laid as chromosomes, gonads, and hormones interact to form primary sexual characteristics. Puberty marks the next major phase, with the activation of secondary sexual traits driven by hormonal surges.

Even after puberty, hormonal changes throughout life continue to influence sexual characteristics. For example:

- Pregnancy in women involves a dramatic increase in estrogen and progesterone, altering body shape and reproductive function.
- Menopause marks the decline of ovarian hormone production, which leads to changes in bone density, skin elasticity, and metabolism.
- Andropause in men involves a gradual decrease in testosterone, affecting muscle mass, energy levels, and libido.

Did You Know?

- *The development of male or female traits depends on genetics and the balance of hormones, which can even override genetic signals in some instances.*
- *Puberty triggers a surge in sex hormones, shaping secondary sexual characteristics like facial hair in boys or breast development in girls.*

Congratulations, You're Expecting a Girl!

Many expectant parents eagerly await learning the sex of their baby, especially mothers, who often feel an intense curiosity about whether they're carrying a boy or a girl. From the early weeks of pregnancy, some parents may rush to the doctor for an ultrasound in hopes of finding out.

But how important is it to know the baby's sex before birth? The answer varies. For some, it's a delightful curiosity; for others, it feels essential. However, many parents express frustration when doctors refuse to disclose the baby's sex until later in the pregnancy.

Why is this the case? Is it truly impossible to determine a baby's sex earlier? The answer is both yes and no. While early ultrasounds can sometimes detect the baby's sex, the results are less accurate, especially if the technician lacks experience. However, the main reason for withholding this information lies not in technical limitations but in ethical considerations.

Cultural and Medical Considerations in Disclosing a Baby's Sex

In many developed countries, disclosing a baby's sex before **24–26 weeks** is discouraged due to concerns about **selective feticide**, the intentional termination of pregnancies based on the baby's sex. This practice is common in certain regions, particularly parts of Asia, where cultural norms often place a higher value on male offspring for reasons like inheritance and lineage.

As immigration brings people from these regions to developed countries, professional medical societies often recommend delaying sex disclosure to reduce the risk of such practices. Although no strict laws regulate this, most progressive doctors adhere to these guidelines to maintain ethical standards. So, if your doctor declines to reveal the baby's sex early, it's not due to a lack of skill or indifference but a commitment to ethical principles.

Exceptions to this practice occur in cases where the baby's sex is medically significant, such as when there is a family history of **sex-linked genetic disorders** or abnormalities in the urinary or reproductive systems.

When Can You Know for Sure if It's a Girl or a Boy?

The earliest determination of a baby's sex can occur at the **eight-cell stage** during **in vitro fertilization (IVF)**. At this stage, **preimplantation genetic testing (PGT)** can assess embryos for genetic disorders and determine their sex before implantation. While this technique is invaluable for identifying inherited diseases linked to the X or Y chromosomes, its use for purely personal reasons, like family balancing, is controversial and criticized.

Another method involves analyzing fetal **DNA (deoxyribonucleic acid)** released into the mother's bloodstream from the placenta early in pregnancy. This DNA can be tested to identify **Y-chromosome markers** indicating a male fetus. If no Y markers are detected, the fetus is presumed female. This technique is non-invasive and increasingly used for early sex determination and screening for chromosomal abnormalities.

Advanced Diagnostic Methods and Safety Considerations

While modern non-invasive techniques are gaining popularity, traditional methods for determining a baby's sex or karyotype (chromosomal makeup) are used in specific medical scenarios. These include:

1. **Chorionic Villus Sampling (CVS)**:
    - Performed between **6–15 weeks** of pregnancy.
    - It involves sampling tissue from the **chorion** (early placenta) to detect genetic abnormalities.

- Risk: ~1 in 100 chance of pregnancy loss.
- Conducted for medical indications only, such as suspected chromosomal disorders.

2. **Amniocentesis**:
   - Performed after **16 weeks** of pregnancy.
   - A small sample of amniotic fluid is taken to analyze fetal chromosomes.
   - Risk: ~1 in 200 chance of pregnancy loss.
   - Often used to diagnose conditions like **Down syndrome**.
3. **Cordocentesis (Umbilical Cord Blood Sampling)**:
   - It is used when the fetus shows signs of anemia or requires an in-utero blood transfusion.
   - It involves sampling blood from the umbilical cord for diagnostic purposes.
   - It is not used solely to determine the baby's sex due to its invasive nature.

These methods carry inherent risks and are recommended only when necessary for diagnosing genetic or chromosomal conditions.

Ultrasound: The Safest Method for Determining Fetal Sex

Ultrasound remains the most common and safest method for determining a baby's sex. However, its accuracy depends on timing and the technician's expertise. During the **11–14-week window**, early genital structures can sometimes be visualized, but errors are common at this stage. By **20 weeks**, the accuracy improves significantly, making it the ideal time for determining the baby's sex.

It's important to note that healthcare providers are generally discouraged from disclosing the baby's sex unless specifically asked by the parents. Statements like "You're having a girl!" without inquiry may infringe upon the parents' right to decide whether they want to know.

For families who do wish to know, the second half of pregnancy is the best time to ask. Knowing the baby's sex allows parents to prepare clothes, nursery décor, and even names. While some cultures discourage early preparations, such superstitions are rare in modern societies.

Did You Know?

- *Early non-invasive blood tests can detect a baby's sex by analyzing fetal DNA in the mother's bloodstream.*
- *Ultrasound is the safest and most common way to determine a baby's sex, with the highest accuracy after 20 weeks of pregnancy.*

Nine Months of Intrauterine Development for a Baby Girl

Does the development and health of female fetuses differ from that of male fetuses? The most significant difference lies in the formation and development of the reproductive organs, although the stages of organ formation in girls and boys are quite similar. But what about overall health?

Pregnancy, birth, and childhood are the three pillars that determine an adult's future health. For those who believe in "destiny," it's important to understand that life in the womb, birth process, and early childhood profoundly impact a person's future. Hidden within these three pillars is another nearly invisible element: the genome (genotype) of the conceived child. Modern Science allows us to study it at the molecular level.

A person's set of genes, arranged in chromosomes, comes from father and mother. This genetic set might seem unchangeable, but the genotype is a dynamic system that is constantly evolving. These changes occur from conception through the end of life, as in any living being carrying encoded information in RNA and DNA. These genetic changes are the basis of evolution, leading to the emergence of thousands of different species of flora and fauna, both past and present. This genetic adaptability is a continuous process, enabling living organisms to adjust to internal and external environmental changes.

Epigenetics and the Factors Influencing Fetal Health

In recent years, **epigenetics**, a science that combines fields like medicine, genetics, biochemistry, biology, ecology, and more, has been rapidly advancing. Epigenetics studies the changes in genes triggered by internal and external environmental factors, a concept scientists call "**genotypic activity**." Interest in genome changes grew through research into disease causes and how early development (including during pregnancy) affects health in adulthood.

Many factors impact the likelihood of a healthy pregnancy and offspring, with the mother's health paramount. The genes a child inherits from both parents determine the structure of cells, tissues, and organs. However, **the mother's health, nutrition, and pregnancy progression are crucial factors affecting the child's well-being**. These factors are further influenced by the external environment in which the mother lives, as it significantly shapes the health of the unborn child. Environmental factors encompass ecological ones (such as pollution, temperature extremes, and noise) and political and social factors (war, economic crises, and instability).

Epigenetics influences fetal health by modifying how genes work without changing their DNA. For example, a mother's stress during pregnancy can affect genes linked to stress response, making a child more sensitive to stress and at higher risk for mood disorders. Similarly, a lack of nutrients like folate or iodine during pregnancy can impact brain development and cognitive abilities. It highlights how a mother's well-being is crucial to a baby's healthy development.

The prevailing attitudes of society toward pregnant women and children, ranging from aggression and indifference to respect for family and motherhood, also affect the developing child. The relationship between the mother, her partner, and other family members is critical. Even if a woman enjoys good health, conflict and violence in her relationship with the future father can lead to serious complications during pregnancy, childbirth, and in the health of the newborn.

Differences in Fetal Reactions Between Girls and Boys

There is a noticeable difference in how male and female fetuses respond to internal and external factors. Initial studies examining the impact of these factors on intrauterine development, survival rates, and newborn health began in the 1980s.

It turns out that pregnancies with male fetuses are more likely to have adverse outcomes, whereas pregnancies with female fetuses generally progress more smoothly. This phenomenon was also observed in research conducted at the start of this century.

Female fetuses develop more slowly than male fetuses, starting from the pre-implantation stage. Male embryos and fetuses are more sensitive to nutritional disruptions, which may arise from placental dysfunction or poor maternal nutrition. Intrauterine growth restriction is more common in male fetuses, and structural or functional abnormalities of the placenta are also more frequent in male pregnancies. Unfortunately, male fetuses experience a higher mortality rate before birth than female fetuses, meaning that pregnancies with boys carry a higher risk of complications.

How can we explain this difference in male and female fetuses' intrauterine development and pregnancy outcomes? Scientists and doctors believe this may be due to the higher nutrient demands of male fetuses. Maternal nutrition and the placenta's capacity to utilize these nutrients from the mother's body are critical factors influencing fetal growth and size.

Summary Table: Key Differences Between Male and Female Fetuses

Factor	Male Fetuses	Female Fetuses
Development Speed	Faster development, especially in early stages.	Slower development starting from the pre-implantation stage.
Placental Efficiency	Placenta operates more efficiently but with lower reserve capacity, making males more vulnerable to stress or malnutrition.	Higher reserve capacity, providing greater resilience to adverse conditions.

Nutritional Sensitivity	More sensitive to nutrient deficiencies; higher risk of intrauterine growth restriction (IUGR).	Better adaptability to nutritional deficits.
Survival Rate	Higher mortality rate before birth due to greater sensitivity to stress and placental dysfunction.	Lower mortality rate before birth; higher survival advantage.
Birth Timing	Born earlier, generally at the same or higher weight relative to females.	Born slightly later; tend to "catch up" on weight before birth.
Body Proportions at Birth	Longer and leaner; larger head circumference.	Rounder bodies; smaller head circumference.
Long-Term Health Implications	Higher risk of cardiovascular diseases if born with low birth weight.	Lower incidence of cardiovascular diseases, indicative of stronger survival mechanisms.

Placenta and Fetal Development: A Genetic Connection

It's essential to remember that the placenta develops from the fertilized egg, sharing the same genetic and chromosomal identity as the fetus. The placenta is a product of the fetus, even though the placenta and embryo formation follow separate paths from the earliest weeks of pregnancy. Therefore, **a healthy conception typically leads to a healthy placenta and fetus**. Conversely, when conception is flawed, abnormalities may be present in both the fetus and the placenta, which may struggle to perform its functions effectively. Such pregnancies are often naturally terminated.

When scientists compared measurements of placentas and fetuses, they discovered a proportional relationship between the two. In other words, smaller babies tend to have smaller placentas. Generally, the placenta's size corresponds to the fetus's size for both girls and boys. However, further comparisons revealed notable differences in body proportions and the weight ratio between the placenta and the fetus in male and female pregnancies. Girls tend to have a higher placenta-to-fetus weight ratio, even though the placenta is smaller.

The Fetal "Programming" of Future Health

The concept of **fetal programming** highlights how adverse conditions during pregnancy, such as nutrient deficiencies or maternal stress, can affect long-term health. For instance:

- Blood flow is redirected to essential organs like the brain and heart at the expense of others, such as the kidneys or liver.
- This redistribution may impair organ development, increasing the risk of diseases like hypertension or metabolic disorders in adulthood.

Animal studies confirm that female fetuses are more resilient to stress and malnutrition than males. However, boys born at term are often stronger and healthier than girls, who tend to have slightly lower birth weights.

Research into how fetal sex influences development and long-term health outcomes is still in its early stages. Male fetuses may be more vulnerable to complications, while female fetuses demonstrate better adaptability, contributing to their survival advantage and longer lifespan.

Did You Know?

- *Male fetuses grow faster but are more sensitive to stress and nutritional deficits, leading to higher risks of complications before birth.*
- *Female fetuses develop more slowly but are more resilient to adverse conditions, contributing to their survival advantage and longer lifespans.*

Girls and Boys: Made from Different Molds?

How different are the development and growth of girls and boys? Parents (and grandparents) with children of both sexes can readily attest that the differences between girls and boys are noticeable from the very first months of life.

We're not just referring to differences in sexual organs or secondary sex characteristics. Physically, girls and boys appear almost identical after birth, apart from their external genitalia. However, as they grow, distinctions emerge in physical traits and in acquiring various skills, responses to their surroundings, interactions with people, behaviors, and more.

What causes these differences? Primarily, it's due to specific brain development differences that begin even in the womb. Whether this unique brain development is genetically programmed or influenced by other factors (like hormones) is unknown. Most likely, it is a combination of factors, including genetics. Specifically, the presence of genes that could be loosely categorized as "male" and "female" genes plays a crucial role in shaping the male and female bodies.

While genetics play a pivotal role, hormones such as testosterone and estrogen exert powerful effects during prenatal development.

Testosterone in male fetuses stimulates the growth of brain regions related to spatial awareness and action-oriented behavior. In contrast, estrogen in female fetuses enhances connectivity between brain regions responsible for verbal communication and emotional regulation.

It's important to note that these biological differences are not fixed. The brain's **neuroplasticity**, its ability to adapt and rewire itself based on experiences, means that environmental factors like parenting, education, and social interactions can amplify or diminish these differences over time.

While scientists from various fields have only recently begun rigorously studying these differences in a scientific context, popular publications on the topic have long been abundant. Advances in science and medicine have made it possible to conduct many of these studies with minimal disruption to children's lives and without risk to their health.

The Practical Importance of Understanding Differences Between Girls and Boys

What is the practical significance of scientifically studying differences between girls and boys? This knowledge, grounded in scientific evidence, helps us better understand the causes and progression of various diseases, as well as the effects of medications and other treatments based on a person's sex. For instance:

- Certain diseases are more common in men than women, and vice versa.
- Medical treatments, including dosages and side effects, may differ significantly depending on biological sex.

Such insights are also invaluable in education. They aid in understanding how children perceive information, allowing teachers to tailor educational programs to account for differences in how boys and girls process information. It helps create individualized learning approaches. Additionally, understanding these differences helps parents interpret their children's behavior more effectively.

For example, girls often excel in verbal tasks early on, benefiting from educational methods emphasizing storytelling and discussions. On the other hand, boys thrive in physical, action-oriented learning environments, which help them focus better and retain information.

People often try to understand themselves and others by analyzing observed differences. Recognizing what is fundamentally determined by biology and sexual differentiation — distinguishing this from myths or misinformation — can help individuals build healthier relationships, feel more comfortable in society, and assist those seeking support and understanding.

This comprehensive table highlights developmental differences between girls and boys across **key developmental factors**. It was created by analyzing multiple research data and publications.

Developmental Factor	**Girls**	**Boys**
Brain Development		
Left Hemisphere (verbal skills)	Develops first and faster—possibly explaining why girls are often more talkative.	Develops more slowly.
Right Hemisphere (spatial skills)	Develops more slowly.	Develops first and faster—possibly explaining better spatial orientation in boys.
Prefrontal Cortex (impulse control, decisions)	Develops by late adolescence (19–20 years); larger in size.	Develops and matures almost until 30 years old.
Amygdala (emotions)	Develops later; starts on the left side; emotions expressed through words; negative emotions move to the cortex.	Develops earlier; starts on the right side; emotions expressed through actions; harder to verbalize negative emotions.

Hippocampus (memory)	Develops earlier; starts on the left; memory for objects and details.	Develops later; starts on the right; memory for images and core meanings.
Corpus Callosum (hemisphere communication)	25% larger by adolescence; hemispheres communicate more effectively.	Hemispheres communicate less than in girls.
Brain Mode	Can switch modes without rest.	Requires rest to recharge and reset.
Brain Use	More cortical processing.	More primitive brain areas are active.
Blood Flow	More blood to the brain's center.	More blood to peripheral brain areas.
Testosterone Influence	Minimal influence on brain development.	Shapes early spatial and motor skills through testosterone surges.
Cognition and Skills		
Spatial Perception	Prefers static objects (e.g., dolls); describes objects better.	Prefers moving objects (e.g., cars, planes); describes locations better.
Speech	Speaks earlier (around 12 months); 100-word vocabulary by 16 months.	Speaks later (13–14 months); 30-word vocabulary by 16 months.

Fine Motor Skills	More refined motor skills by age 6 (e.g., drawing, writing).	Develops purposeful gross motor skills by age 4 (e.g., jumping, running).
Attention Focus	More on faces and static objects; uses warm colors.	More on movement; uses cool colors.
Information Processing	Better with verbal and auditory cues.	Better with tactile and visual cues.
Self-Assessment	Tends to underestimate own abilities.	Tends to overestimate own abilities.
Problem-Solving	Lower risk tolerance; prefers diplomatic solutions.	Higher risk tolerance; more impulsive solutions.
Multitasking	Can handle multiple tasks and switch attention easily.	Prefers sequential tasks; slower at switching attention.
Fight-or-Flight Response (adrenaline)	Less frequent.	More frequent.
Friendship/Attachment Response (oxytocin)	Dominant; calming response.	Less common.
Reactions to General Statements	Tends to feel irritated.	Tends to react with anger.
Physical Development		
Growth Patterns	Grow faster during early childhood but	Growth spurts occur later but are typically

	slower after puberty starts.	more pronounced.
Bone Density and Muscle Mass	Develop stronger bone density earlier; less muscle mass and higher fat percentage.	Greater muscle mass and lean body composition; longer bone growth during adolescence.
Puberty Onset	Begins earlier (8–13 years) with breast development and menstruation.	Begins later (9–14 years) with testicular enlargement and voice deepening.
Hormonal Regulation		
Estrogen vs. Testosterone	Estrogen promotes skeletal maturation and fat distribution.	Testosterone drives muscle growth and aggressive behaviors.
Cortisol (Stress Hormone)	Higher cortisol sensitivity; prone to anxiety under stress.	Less prone to anxiety but more physical frustration under stress.
Social Skills		
Recognizing Emotions	Better at reading facial expressions and emotional cues.	Less attentive to others' emotional states.
Friendship	Based on personality; conversation-focused; avoids hierarchy.	Based on shared interests; conversations considered secondary;

		accepts hierarchy.
Communication Style	Prefers face-to-face communication.	Prefers shoulder-to-shoulder interaction.
Attachment	Forms deeper emotional bonds through shared experiences.	Forms bonds through shared activities or interests.
Sensory Sensitivity		
Hearing	More sensitive; better at distinguishing tone and volume.	More issues recognizing audio cues.
Vision	Better at seeing close, static objects; better memory for color and shades.	Better at assessing distant, moving objects; less focus on color.
Touch	Prefers observing and tactile precision.	Prefers exploring through active touch.
Pain Sensitivity	Greater sensitivity to pain; may vocalize discomfort.	Less sensitive to pain; often suppresses signs of discomfort.
Play Behavior and Preferences		
Play Style	Prefers collaborative role-playing activities (e.g., "family").	Prefers rough-and-tumble play and competitive games.
Caution vs. Risk	More cautious; avoids risky	More adventurous;

	physical behaviors.	prone to physical risk-taking.
Feelings and Emotions		
Emotional Expression	Verbally expressive; more comfortable sharing feelings.	Actions often express complex emotions; less comfortable discussing feelings.
Fear Response	Tends to feel weak or helpless in fear-inducing situations.	Tends to feel strong or excited in response to fear.
Aggression	Rarely used in play.	Commonly expressed in play.
Crying	Cries more during adolescence.	Cries more between 6 months and preschool.
Separation Anxiety	Adjusts more easily.	Experiences more difficulty.
Stress Handling	Struggles more; learning often impacted by stress.	Manages stress better; may exhibit more outward frustration.
Learning and Schooling		
Preschool Adaptation	Adapts more easily.	75% face adaptation challenges.
Math	Requires more focus but benefits	Solves problems faster but often with less

	from structured learning.	attention to detail.
Reading	Reads earlier, prefers fictional stories.	Lags 1–1.5 years behind; prefers factual, technical reading.
Words vs. Images	Learns better through text or sound.	Learns better through visuals and diagrams.
Task Switching	Faster.	Slower.
Study Posture	Learns best seated and relaxed.	Learns best standing or actively engaged.
Group Size	Performs better in small groups (2–4 people).	Prefers larger groups but is easily distracted.
Homework	Tends to be meticulous, completing tasks fully.	Often less precise; may not finish tasks.
Problem-Solving Style	Prefers face-to-face problem-solving.	Prefers side-by-side problem-solving.
Learning Motivation	Believes effort is key to success.	Believes innate abilities are key to success.
Grades	Around 30% satisfactory or average grades.	Around 70% satisfactory or average grades.
Teacher Influence	More likely to seek help; values teacher friendships.	Influenced but dislikes overly talkative teachers; less likely to seek help.

Classroom Behavior	Accounts for 20% of behavior issues; often seen as a behavioral "gold standard."	Accounts for 80% of behavior issues; male behavior often misinterpreted as female-like deficits.
Attention and Learning Disorders		
Attention Deficit and ADHD	Less common, with better focus.	More common, issues with attention retention.
Learning Disorders	30% of cases.	70% of cases.
Dyslexia	Less common.	More common.
Dysgraphia/Dyspraxia	More accurate in writing and grammar.	Greater challenges with spelling and expressing thoughts in writing.
School Dropout Rate	20% of dropouts, but fewer leave school early.	

Naturally, these are just some general differences between girls and boys. It's important to remember that many women may identify with traits commonly associated with men, and likewise, many men may exhibit characteristics traditionally considered feminine. These overlaps highlight the diversity and complexity of individual personalities and behaviors.

While most of these differences are rooted in genetics and brain development, the environment also plays a pivotal role in shaping a child's growth. Factors such as living conditions, nutrition, and especially the social environment, as well as the people who frequently interact with and influence the child, profoundly impact their development.

In newborns and infants, gender-related differences are minimal. Over time, "masculine" and "feminine" traits emerge through interactions with close family members, caregivers, and society. Since the dawn of civilization, cultural expectations have shaped the upbringing of girls and boys, and many of these expectations persist today. As a result, the development of men and women often mirrors society's longstanding values and traditions. Even in single-parent families, children tend to adopt traits associated with their biological gender by observing and imitating others in their community.

However, it's vital to respect a child's individuality.

Children should not be molded into puppets, dolls, or copies of their parents, nor should they be forced to conform to rigid standards based on parental preferences or societal stereotypes. Instead, parents should observe and nurture their child's natural interests, strengths, and passions.

In today's evolving world, we are also beginning to recognize that gender identity may extend beyond traditional concepts of "male" and "female." While biological differences are undeniable, every child is unique, and a combination of nature and nurture shapes their identity. Embracing this diversity allows parents to provide the support and understanding every child deserves.

Understanding the psychophysiological differences between genders can help parents better appreciate and nurture their children's unique qualities. This knowledge fosters healthier relationships between parents and children and deepens understanding and harmony within families and couples.

Please encourage your child to explore their individuality while respecting their natural development. Celebrate their strengths, support their challenges, and, most importantly, let them grow into the best version of themselves. By embracing these principles, we can create a future where children feel confident, understood, and deeply valued for who they are.

Did You Know?

- *Girls tend to develop verbal skills earlier, while boys often excel in spatial tasks, showcasing distinct brain development patterns.*
- *Brain neuroplasticity means that parenting, education, and social interactions can reshape and balance these natural differences over time.*

What Affects a Girl's Health?

Even without a medical background, most readers would agree that many factors influence the health of both girls and boys. However, parental and societal attitudes toward girls, including the level of care provided, often differ from those toward boys. Many people perceive girls as more delicate and, therefore, more susceptible to illness. Studies show that parents, particularly mothers, tend to spend more time with girls from birth than with boys.

But are girls truly weaker and less healthy than boys? While girls are typically born with lower birth weights and may experience more complications during the early neonatal period, their health often improves rapidly, and their growth and development align with those of boys when proper care is provided. Girls are frequently less fussy (unless spoiled by excessive attention) and more patient, suggesting that they should not automatically be considered the "weaker" sex.

Interestingly, girls and women can endure prolonged moderate physical activity with less harm to their health than boys and men. However, brief, intense physical exertion is more challenging for the female body. This observation highlights differences in biological endurance rather than physical strength.

Biopsychosocial Model: A Holistic Perspective on Health

Examining the broader determinants of human health is crucial to understanding the factors affecting girls' health. In 1977, American psychiatrist George Engel introduced a groundbreaking concept, the biopsychosocial model, in the journal *Science*. This model categorized health determinants into three interconnected domains:

1. **Biological**: Heredity, genetic traits, sex, and physical condition.

2. **Psychological**: Thoughts, emotions, and behaviors.
3. **Social**: Socioeconomic factors, environment, culture, and societal norms.

This comprehensive model emphasized the interplay between internal and external factors influencing health and illness. Engel's work shifted the mindset of many doctors, encouraging a view of the patient as a whole rather than focusing narrowly on isolated organs or symptoms.

Today, Engel's model remains relevant, particularly in pediatric care. For parents, understanding the biopsychosocial model offers profound insights into the factors shaping their child's well-being. This approach encourages a shift from isolated observations of symptoms to a comprehensive view that considers physical, emotional, and environmental influences.

All processes in the human body occur at the molecular level, driven by intricate chemical reactions that produce or absorb energy and create essential substances. Healthy cell structures form the foundation for tissues, which build functioning organs. These organs rely on biochemical reactions to carry out genetic instructions encoded in DNA. The nervous system, especially the brain, is pivotal in coordinating these processes, ensuring harmony across all systems.

By applying Engel's biopsychosocial model, parents can better understand how interconnected factors affect their children and work toward fostering balance in their development.

Other Models of Health and Development

While Engel's biopsychosocial model remains a cornerstone for understanding health, additional frameworks have emerged to deepen our insights into the factors that influence health, particularly in children. These modern models emphasize the intricate interplay of biological, behavioral, and environmental factors, broadening how we view health and development.

The Ecological Systems Theory (Bronfenbrenner, 1979)

The Ecological Systems Theory, created by a renowned American developmental psychologist, Urie Bronfenbrenner, provides a comprehensive perspective on child development, emphasizing that multiple interconnected systems influence a child's growth. Each of these layers interacts with and shapes the others, creating a dynamic environment for development:

- **Microsystem**: The child's immediate environment, such as family, school, peers, and direct interactions with caregivers. These close relationships have the most immediate and significant impact on the child's well-being.
- **Mesosystem**: The connections between microsystems, such as the relationship between parents and teachers or between siblings and friends. Positive mesosystem interactions reinforce a child's sense of stability and support.
- **Exosystem**: Indirect environments that affect the child, such as a parent's workplace or neighborhood conditions. Although the child is not directly involved, these factors influence the family's dynamics and resources.
- **Macrosystem**: Broader societal and cultural influences, including societal norms, laws, policies, and values. These shape the framework within which all other systems operate.
- **Chronosystem**: The dimension of time, accounting for life transitions (e.g., a family move, parental divorce) and historical or generational events that impact development, such as a global pandemic or economic crisis.

This theory highlights how a child's development is not isolated but shaped by the interactions within and between these systems. Understanding these layers allows parents, educators, and healthcare providers to address challenges in a child's environment effectively.

The Social Determinants of Health (WHO, 2008)

The Social Determinants of Health framework, introduced by the World Health Organization, underscores how societal and environmental factors profoundly influence health outcomes. This model identifies key determinants that can either promote or hinder a person's health:

- **Access to healthcare**: The availability and affordability of quality healthcare services directly impact physical and mental well-being.
- **Education and literacy**: Higher levels of education improve health literacy, enabling individuals to make informed decisions about their health.
- **Economic stability**: Stable income and financial security reduce stress and allow families to access nutritious food, safe housing, and healthcare.
- **Housing and living conditions**: Clean, safe, and stable housing is a foundation for good health. Overcrowding or unsafe environments can lead to physical and mental health challenges.
- **Social support and inclusion**: Strong social networks and a sense of community improve emotional resilience and reduce the risk of isolation-related health issues.

This model highlights the structural and systemic influences on health, emphasizing the need to address inequalities to ensure all children have an equal chance at a healthy life.

The Life Course Model (1995)

The Life Course Model, popularized by Dr. Clyde Hertzman and other researchers, views health as a dynamic process shaped by experiences throughout life, beginning even before birth. It draws heavily on findings from David Barker's "fetal origins of adult disease" hypothesis. Key principles include:

- **Early life experiences lay the foundation for future health**: Prenatal care, infant nutrition, and early childhood interactions significantly impact long-term well-being. For example, maternal stress or malnutrition during pregnancy can program a child's health trajectory.

- **Adverse Childhood Events (ACEs) have lasting effects**: Events such as abuse, neglect, or family instability can increase the risk of chronic diseases, mental health disorders, and lower socioeconomic outcomes later in life.
- **Health behaviors and risks accumulate over time**: Habits, environmental exposures, and life choices influence health outcomes. Positive behaviors, such as exercise and balanced nutrition, reinforce resilience, while negative factors, such as smoking or poor diet, exacerbate risks.

This model reinforces the importance of early intervention and sustained support throughout a person's life. Recognizing health as cumulative helps parents and caregivers nurture healthy behaviors and minimize risk factors from the earliest stages of life.

Health is not a fixed state, but an evolving journey shaped by a complex web of interrelated factors. From a child's immediate family to broader societal structures, from genetic inheritance to environmental exposures, every layer contributes to shaping their health and development. These influences interact continuously, creating a dynamic interplay that changes over time.

For parents, understanding these models provides a roadmap for creating environments that nurture physical, emotional, and social well-being. By addressing not only biological needs but also psychological and societal influences, we can lay the foundation for healthier outcomes, not just for children today but for future generations.

Humans are inherently social beings, relying on connections with family, community, and society for survival and growth. These relationships profoundly shape an individual's worldview, attitudes toward health, and even physical experiences. The social environment, including family dynamics and societal norms, can significantly impact a child's development.

Environmental conditions such as climate, living standards, and access to healthcare also play a pivotal role in determining health outcomes. Socioeconomic factors significantly influence a family's ability to provide balanced nutrition, access medical care, and create a safe, nurturing environment. For example, families in low-income neighborhoods may face challenges like overcrowded housing, limited access to quality education, and environmental hazards, all of which can affect a child's health and development.

For children, especially girls, the quality of these external factors directly impacts their physical and emotional development. Societal attitudes toward girls' abilities and roles can shape how they perceive themselves and their health, influencing their confidence, self-care habits, and long-term well-being. Recognizing these influences empowers parents to create positive environments for their daughters, fostering resilience and self-worth.

Focus on Girls: Overcoming Unique Challenges

Girls face societal challenges that directly or indirectly influence their health and well-being. These challenges often stem from cultural norms and expectations that shape how girls perceive themselves and their place in the world.

One notable issue is **stereotypes about physical activity**. Cultural attitudes, even in modern societies, may discourage girls from participating in sports or physical challenges, reinforcing the false belief that such activities are "unfeminine." Yet, regular exercise is vital for a girl's physical and mental health, improving cardiovascular fitness, strength, and emotional resilience. Encouraging girls to break free from these stereotypes and embrace physical activities not only boosts their self-esteem but also establishes lifelong habits of well-being.

Another significant challenge is **body image pressure**. Research reveals that girls as young as eight years old can begin developing concerns about their appearance due to societal beauty standards. These unrealistic ideals often lead to unhealthy behaviors, such as restrictive eating or overexercising, in an attempt to conform. Parents play a crucial role in fostering a positive body image by emphasizing the value of health over appearance and teaching their daughters to appreciate their unique qualities. Modeling self-acceptance and avoiding negative comments about weight or appearance are critical strategies for helping girls build confidence.

Finally, **access to education and healthcare** remains an issue for many girls globally. In some regions, girls face significant barriers to receiving quality education or medical care, often due to gender biases or economic constraints. Limited access to these resources deprives girls of the opportunity to thrive, both physically and mentally. Advocating for equitable access to education and healthcare is essential for ensuring their well-being and helping them realize their full potential.

By addressing these unique challenges, parents can empower their daughters to navigate societal pressures while fostering confidence, resilience, and a strong sense of self-worth.

Insights from Recent Research

Scientific research highlights the profound impact that parental involvement and societal influences have on girls' mental and physical health outcomes:

- **Mental health resilience**: A 2022 study revealed that daughters who share strong emotional bonds with their parents are 40% less likely to experience anxiety and depression during adolescence. A key protective factor was parental validation of their daughters' emotions, which helped them develop emotional security and self-esteem.
- **Long-term health habits**: Girls whose parents actively encourage participation in physical activity are twice as likely to maintain regular exercise habits into adulthood as

those who do not receive such encouragement. It underscores the importance of early exposure to sports and fitness in shaping lifelong behaviors.

- **Impact of early interventions**: A 2020 review found that parents who proactively address societal biases, such as gender stereotypes, significantly boost their daughters' self-efficacy and career aspirations. Challenging these biases equips girls with the confidence to pursue their goals without feeling constrained by outdated expectations.

By applying these research findings, parents can take practical steps to optimize their daughters' health and development. Providing emotional support, encouraging active lifestyles, and addressing societal biases benefit girls during childhood and lay the groundwork for their long-term well-being and success.

Parents as the First Line of Care

Parents are central to ensuring their child's growth, development, and overall health. While pediatricians play a vital role in identifying and addressing health concerns, parents witness their child's daily life and subtle changes that might go unnoticed in a clinical setting. Their attentiveness often forms the first line of defense against potential health issues.

Of course, not all parents are equally engaged, and some may neglect their children's needs. However, this book was written for mothers and fathers who deeply care about their children's well-being. These parents prioritize proper nutrition and a healthy environment and respect each family member, whether daughter, son, or partner, as a unique individual with an inner world influenced by external circumstances.

For parents, this means being proactive, observant, and willing to adapt. By fostering open communication, encouraging healthy habits, and providing emotional support, parents can empower their children to thrive in a complex and ever-changing world.

Practical Steps for Parents

Parents can take several steps to foster holistic health in their children:

1. **Create stress-free routines**: Consistent daily schedules with adequate time for sleep, meals, and play help regulate children's emotions and reduce stress.
2. **Encourage hobbies and activities**: Girls benefit significantly from activities that build self-confidence and resilience, such as sports, arts, or problem-solving games. These also challenge stereotypes about their capabilities.
3. **Provide a balanced diet**: Proper nutrition is critical for cognitive and physical development. Involve children in meal planning to teach them about healthy eating habits.
4. **Promote open communication**: Encourage your child to openly share their thoughts and feelings. Research shows that strong parental support reduces the risk of anxiety and depression, especially in adolescent girls.
5. **Be a role model**: Demonstrate healthy habits and attitudes toward your health. Children are more likely to adopt behaviors they see modeled by their parents.

Ultimately, the factors that influence a girl's health are the same as those affecting boys, all children, and every individual. What matters most is the ability to nurture a child holistically, addressing physical, emotional, and social needs while recognizing the unique qualities that make each person special.

Understanding and acting upon these interconnected factors can create a stronger foundation for lifelong health and well-being. By embracing this holistic perspective, parents and caregivers can help ensure that every child, regardless of gender, has the opportunity to flourish and reach their full potential.

Did You Know?

- *Urie Bronfenbrenner's Ecological Systems Theory inspired the design of the U.S. Head Start Program. This program helps children from low-income families by integrating education, nutrition, and health services, reflecting Bronfenbrenner's belief in addressing a child's development through a multi-layered support system.*
- *The Life Course Model traces a child's health journey back to conditions in the womb. Maternal nutrition, stress, and early-life events have a profound impact on lifelong health outcomes, linking fetal experiences to adult diseases.*

Stages of Development and Their Characteristics

Children are dynamic, living systems undergoing continuous, rapid transformations that make comparisons to adult physiological processes almost impossible. Consider the extraordinary transformation from a single fertilized egg into a 3.5-kilogram baby in just nine months of pregnancy! Although growth slows slightly after birth, the first year of life is still marked by remarkable milestones. **Infants typically double their birth weight and increase their length by about one and a half times.**

From birth through adolescence and until the completion of puberty, the body undergoes continual transformations, albeit at slower rates. Plotting these changes on a graph would form a curve resembling an inverse geometric progression.

Despite this slowing, children remain in a constant state of flux. Their bodies are highly dynamic, with rapid growth, development, and recovery capabilities that far exceed those of adults. Illnesses may appear and progress more quickly in children, but their remarkable recovery ability reflects their faster metabolic rates, better tissue blood flow, and higher fluid content.

Understanding the Rapid Changes in Child Development

From birth to approximately 21–22 years, a child's body undergoes rapid transformations defining growth and development. This dynamism explains why illnesses in children may arise and progress differently than in adults. However, the same dynamism also equips children with a unique capacity for recovery, highlighting the resilience of the developing body.

Experts have divided childhood and adolescence into distinct stages and benchmarks for assessing developmental milestones. While chronological age may not always align with biological age, especially in cases such as premature births, these categories provide a practical framework for understanding growth patterns.

Numerous theories on child development exist, encompassing ecological, psychoanalytic, and cognitive perspectives. However, age-based classifications remain the most practical tools for pediatric care. They help healthcare providers and parents assess whether children are meeting developmental milestones and identify potential issues.

Modern pediatrics often evaluates a child's development starting from the fetal period, which averages 280 days. This prenatal stage is crucial, as it establishes the foundation for long-term health. Pediatricians frequently request detailed pregnancy histories, including test results and ultrasound findings, to better understand a child's early development.

Life begins at conception, not birth. Recognizing this is vital for ensuring proper care and avoiding harm during prenatal development. After birth, the child transitions to a new external environment, where continued growth and development unfold in distinct stages:

- **0–1 year**: Newborn and infancy period, divided into:
    - 0–2 months
    - 2–6 months
    - 6–12 months
- **1–3 years**: Early preschool age, including:
    - 12–18 months
    - 18–24 months
    - 24–36 months
- **3–6 years**: Preschool period.
- **6–12 years**: School age, including early puberty (8–12 years).
- **12–20 (21) years**: Adolescent period.

These stages align with developmental theories used by healthcare providers to assess intellectual, psychosocial, and motor skills. However, parents' primary concern during doctor visits often concerns one question: "Is my child healthy?"

Parents often evaluate growth and health through personal observations, relying on their knowledge and experiences. Having access to reliable, evidence-based resources written by medical professionals is invaluable. Unfortunately, many parents rely on anecdotal advice rather than authoritative sources. Preparing for pregnancy and child-rearing well in advance can significantly ease the challenges of parenthood.

Growth Patterns in Boys and Girls

Growth charts reveal that boys' height slightly surpasses girls' until around age 10–11. During early puberty, however, girls experience a growth spurt, briefly outpacing boys in height. By age 14, boys' growth accelerates significantly, and they generally outgrow girls as their growth continues for a more extended period. After birth, growth rates naturally slow but accelerate again during puberty. Girls reach their peak growth velocity 2–3 years earlier than boys, though boys ultimately experience more significant overall height increases.

Weight gain generally parallels height growth. Girls hit their peak weight gain earlier than boys during adolescence. Boys later experience rapid weight increases, primarily driven by muscle mass expansion and height growth.

Genetics significantly influence body structure and metabolic rates. For instance, tall, slim parents often have children with similar traits. However, lifestyle factors, particularly diet and physical activity, play an equally critical role. In modern societies with diets high in refined sugars and fats and reduced physical activity, childhood obesity rates are increasing alarmingly.

Two periods in a child's life stand out due to their dynamic changes: infancy (up to 1 year) and adolescence (ages 11–20).

- **Infancy**: Though hormonally inactive, this phase is marked by rapid physical growth, sensory development, and adaptation to life outside the womb. Cognitive and motor milestones develop rapidly during this time.

- **Adolescence** is characterized by hormonal activity, accelerated growth, sexual maturation, and evolving self-awareness ("Ego"). It brings significant emotional and psychological changes shaped by emerging independence and identity formation.

While sexual development will be explored in a separate chapter, recent studies indicate that secondary sexual characteristics (e.g., breast development, external genital changes, body hair) are influenced not only by age but also by gender and ethnicity. Parents and healthcare providers must consider these factors when assessing adolescent development.

Did You Know?

- *Infants typically double their birth weight within the first year of life. This rapid growth highlights the importance of proper nutrition during infancy.*
- *Genetics largely determine a child's height, but diet and exercise significantly impact weight. Encouraging healthy eating and physical activity helps mitigate genetic predispositions.*

Health in the First Years of Life (Birth to 2 Years)

The first two years of life are a period of rapid and remarkable growth, laying the foundation for a child's lifelong health and development. During this critical stage, physical, cognitive, and emotional milestones are achieved at an unprecedented pace, making it essential for caregivers to prioritize the child's well-being and adapt to their evolving needs.

Physically, infants experience exponential growth, doubling their birth weight by six months and tripling it by their first birthday.

Height increases rapidly, bones strengthen, and the nervous system develops, enabling significant advancements in motor skills. From the initial reflex-driven movements of a newborn to a toddler's first steps, this period is marked by continuous progress. Proper nutrition, particularly breastfeeding or formula feeding in infancy and the gradual introduction of solid foods, is crucial in supporting this growth.

Cognitively, the first two years are a time of intense brain development.

Neural connections are formed at an extraordinary rate, influenced by sensory experiences, interaction with caregivers, and exploration of the environment. Babies begin to recognize familiar faces, respond to voices, and develop the ability to understand and communicate their needs. Encouraging interaction through touch, eye contact, and speech fosters intellectual and emotional growth, laying the groundwork for language and social skills.

Emotionally and socially, the first years of life are defined by forming secure attachments.

The bond between a caregiver and child is the foundation for emotional regulation, trust, and relationships later in life. Consistent care, affection, and responsiveness to a baby's needs help establish safety and comfort.

During this period, health care focuses on preventive measures and monitoring **developmental milestones**. Routine pediatric check-ups, vaccinations, and screenings ensure potential health issues are identified early and promptly addressed. Parents and caregivers must also prioritize hygiene, safe sleep practices, and accident prevention to protect the child from illness and injury.

The first two years are also a time of immense learning for caregivers as they adapt to the demands of nurturing a growing child. Understanding the importance of early health interventions, creating a supportive environment, and fostering a loving relationship are essential for promoting the child's physical, emotional, and cognitive well-being.

In this critical stage of life, every interaction and care decision build a strong foundation for the child's future. We equip them with the tools they need to grow, thrive, and reach their full potential by meeting their basic needs and responding to their developmental milestones.

Did you know?

- *During the first year of life, a baby's brain doubles in size, forming over a million new neural connections every second. Sensory experiences, interactions with caregivers, and a stimulating environment heavily influence these rapid developments.*
- *By the age of two, children typically reach about half their adult height and triple their birth weight, showcasing the remarkable pace of physical growth in the early years of life.*

"Strange" Phenomena in Newborns

The first days and weeks after birth are often filled with stress from multiple sources: the physical exhaustion of childbirth, emotional fluctuations, and the mother's adjustment to postpartum changes, usually accompanied by discomfort and complaints. Adding to this is the need to establish a new daily routine centered around the newborn's needs. The demands of caring for a new family member can feel overwhelming, especially for first-time parents. Anxiety about the baby's health often arises, mainly when the infant cries frequently, develops a fever, experiences bloating, or has prolonged jaundice. Unfortunately, the overinvolvement of healthcare providers through frequent interventions and instructions can sometimes amplify rather than reduce parental stress.

- ***The First Few Weeks: A Dual Adaptation Process***

The first three weeks after birth are often the most challenging for both parents and newborns. This period marks a time of significant adaptation: the newborn must adjust to life outside the womb while parents adapt to meet the constant needs of their baby. During these weeks, wakefulness, feeding, and sleep routines begin to emerge. Establishing balance is essential; allowing the baby's needs to dominate every aspect of the family's schedule can lead to parental exhaustion. Instead, parents should gently guide their child into a rhythm that accommodates the newborn's needs and the family's well-being.

Among the many changes parents observe in their newborn during this period are certain "strange" phenomena linked to hormonal influences, such as vaginal discharge, breast swelling, and even discharge from the nipples. Though often discussed in pediatric texts, these occurrences are typically explained in oversimplified terms. It is widely stated that maternal estrogens pass into the baby's bloodstream during pregnancy, and their residual presence after birth causes these changes. While partially accurate, this explanation cannot fully capture these processes' complexity.

To provide a more precise understanding, let us delve into the hormonal environment of pregnancy and the unique dynamics at play in the newborn's body during the first days and weeks of life.

- ***Understanding Hormonal Dynamics During Pregnancy***

Pregnancy is a unique physiological state where maternal ovarian activity temporarily ceases. By the 7th or 8th week of pregnancy, the mother's ovaries effectively enter a state of "physiological menopause," becoming inactive for the duration of the pregnancy. Ovulation and menstrual cycles halt entirely as the placenta assumes full responsibility for hormone production.

After conception, the corpus luteum, a structure formed in the ovary after ovulation, initially produces progesterone, which is essential for maintaining the early stages of pregnancy. However, its role is short-lived. Once implantation occurs and the placenta begins to develop, it takes over progesterone production, rendering the corpus luteum unnecessary by the end of the first trimester.

The placenta is not just a provider of nutrients but also a robust endocrine organ that produces vast quantities of steroid hormones, including progesterone, estrogens, and androgens. These hormones are critical for the mother and the developing fetus, facilitating fetal growth and ensuring pregnancy stability. Hormone concentrations in the fetal environment, comprising amniotic fluid, fetal tissues, and blood, are significantly higher than in the mother's blood, immersing the fetus in a unique hormonal "bath."

For example:

- **Estradiol**, the dominant estrogen in adult women, is also present in high levels during pregnancy. Its concentration in maternal blood is roughly 2.5 times higher than in the fetus.
- **Estriol**, another type of estrogen, is produced almost exclusively by the placenta. Its levels in the fetus are four times higher than in the mother, underscoring the

independence of fetal hormone synthesis from maternal contributions.

By the end of pregnancy, nearly all steroid hormones in the fetal system are synthesized by the placenta and fetal tissues themselves.

While maternal hormonal imbalances in early pregnancy may influence development, the fetus and placenta primarily operate independently in the later stages.

- ***Post-Birth Hormonal Shifts in Newborns***

At birth, the newborn is abruptly disconnected from the placenta, its primary source of steroid hormones. Despite this disconnection, hormone levels in the baby's blood remain extraordinarily high immediately after delivery, a legacy of the fetal environment. Over the first 24 hours, these hormones begin to break down and are excreted. The hormone metabolism and excretion process are most intense in the initial days of life, leading to a rapid decline in concentrations.

For instance:

- Progesterone levels in umbilical cord blood range from 440 to 2000 ng/mL, averaging around 1030 ng/mL. By the end of the first day, levels drop to approximately 20 ng/mL, and by the third day, they stabilize at around eight ng/mL.
- Estriol, another key hormone, also decreases significantly within days of birth.

These hormonal fluctuations manifest in several physical changes that often alarm parents, including:

- Swelling of the labia and hymen in girls.
- Vaginal discharge, sometimes blood-tinged (often likened to a "mini period").
- Breast swelling and nipple discharge (commonly called "witch's milk") in both sexes.

- ***Parental Reassurance: What's Normal?***

Parents should understand that these phenomena are every day and transient. They reflect the body's adjustment to the loss of placental hormones and do not indicate any underlying health issue.

***Common Signs That Are Normal*:**

- **Swelling:** Temporary enlargement of the labia, hymen, or breasts typically resolves within weeks.
- **Discharge:** Clear, milky, or blood-tinged vaginal discharge in girls is harmless and usually lasts a few days.
- **Nipple Discharge:** Small amounts of milky secretion from the nipples in boys or girls are normal and self-limiting.

***When to Seek Medical Advice*:**

- Symptoms persist beyond six weeks.
- Signs of infection, such as fever, redness, or pus, accompany these changes.
- Additional concerning symptoms, such as poor feeding or lethargy, are observed.

While these hormonal phenomena may initially seem concerning, they are a natural part of the newborn's adaptation to life outside the womb. By understanding the underlying processes, parents can feel reassured and confident in supporting their baby during this transitional phase. If there are lingering concerns, consulting with a pediatrician can provide further guidance and peace of mind.

Did You Know?

- *Breast swelling in newborns, sometimes called "witch's milk," is a natural response to hormonal changes, not a cause for concern.*
- *The placenta produces far more hormones during pregnancy than a woman's ovaries do at any other time.*

Feeding and Nutrition for Infants

Proper nutrition during the first year of life is critical for an infant's growth, development, and long-term health. As the fastest period of physical and cognitive growth, infancy demands a carefully planned and responsive approach to feeding. From breastfeeding or formula feeding in the early months to the introduction of solid foods later in the first year, parents and caregivers play a pivotal role in shaping a healthy nutritional foundation.

However, I want to clarify that the purpose of this book is not to provide an exhaustive description of the postpartum period or lactation (a topic I have covered in another book). Nor is it intended to serve as a detailed pediatrics manual or a comprehensive guide on feeding and caring for a child during the first year of life (many excellent books by other authors already exist on this subject). For this reason, I will not focus too heavily on newborn and infant nutrition. Instead, I will summarize key knowledge and insights in a concise overview of the most essential points.

Breast milk is universally recognized as the gold standard in infant nutrition.

It provides a perfectly balanced composition of nutrients, antibodies, and enzymes tailored to meet an infant's needs. Beyond nourishment, breastfeeding fosters a deep emotional bond between the mother and baby, offering comfort, security, and physical closeness.

The World Health Organization (WHO) and many pediatric associations recommend exclusive breastfeeding for the first six months of life. Exclusive breastfeeding means no other foods or liquids are introduced; only breast milk supplies all the water, calories, and nutrients the baby requires. Of course, not all doctors, caregivers, and parents agree with such WHO recommendations, believing they are primarily designed for regions of the world where children face hunger and maternal milk is often the only available source of nutrition.

Breastfeeding offers numerous health benefits, including:

- **Immune Protection**: Antibodies in breast milk protect against infections, such as respiratory illnesses, diarrhea, and ear infections.
- **Digestive Health**: Breast milk is easily digested, reducing the likelihood of colic, constipation, and gastroesophageal reflux.
- **Chronic Disease Prevention**: Breastfeeding has been associated with lower risks of asthma, allergies, obesity, and type 2 diabetes later in life.

However, breastfeeding is not always straightforward for every mother. Challenges such as latching difficulties, insufficient milk supply, or maternal health conditions may arise. Support from healthcare professionals, lactation consultants, and peer support groups can help mothers navigate these issues successfully. Infant formula provides a safe and nutritious alternative for mothers who cannot or choose not to breastfeed.

Infant formula is specifically designed to mimic the composition of breast milk, providing essential nutrients for growth and development.

While it cannot replicate breast milk's antibodies or living components, modern formulas are nutritionally complete and ensure healthy development when prepared and used correctly. Parents should consult their pediatrician when choosing a formula, particularly if the infant has specific needs, such as lactose intolerance or milk protein allergies. Standard formulas are cow's milk-based, with modifications to make them digestible for infants. Alternatives include soy-based formulas, hydrolyzed protein formulas for sensitive digestion, or specialized options for premature babies or those with metabolic disorders.

Most infants are developmentally ready to begin transitioning to solid foods around six months of age. This phase, known as **complementary feeding**, introduces textures and flavors that expand an infant's palate while continuing to provide breast milk or formula as the primary source of nutrition.

Signs of readiness for solids include:

- Sitting up with minimal support.
- Good head and neck control.
- Showing interest in food, such as reaching for or mimicking eating behaviors.
- Diminished tongue-thrust reflex, allowing them to swallow solids without pushing them out.

The introduction of solid foods should be gradual and thoughtful. Start with single-ingredient, iron-rich options such as fortified cereals, pureed meats, or lentils. Pureed vegetables and fruits can follow, ensuring a variety of nutrients. There are no differences in the approach to introducing solid foods based on the child's gender.

Key principles for introducing solids:

- Iron First: Iron is vital for brain development and growth, and infants' natural stores begin to deplete around six months. Iron-fortified cereals, pureed meats, and legumes should be prioritized.
- One at a Time: Introduce one new food every 3–5 days to monitor for potential allergies or sensitivities. Based on pediatric recommendations, common allergens such as eggs, peanuts, or fish can be introduced early in small amounts.
- Textures and Progression: Start with smooth purees and gradually progress to mashed and finger foods as chewing skills develop.

While early exposure to potential allergens can reduce the likelihood of developing allergies, certain foods should be avoided entirely during the first year:

- Honey: Risk of infant botulism.
- Cow's Milk: Unsuitable as a primary drink until after 12 months due to its low iron content and risk of interfering with nutrient absorption.

- Choking Hazards: Small, solid, or sticky foods such as whole nuts, popcorn, or large raw vegetables.
- Added Sugars and Salt: Avoid processed foods high in sugar or salt, as these can strain immature kidneys and contribute to unhealthy eating habits.

Feeding during infancy is not only about nourishment; it is an opportunity to build trust and respond to a child's cues.

Responsive feeding encourages caregivers to recognize hunger and satiety signals rather than adhering to rigid schedules. This approach helps prevent overfeeding or underfeeding while fostering a positive relationship with food.

Did you know?

- *Breast milk is universally recognized as the gold standard in infant nutrition. It provides a perfect balance of nutrients, antibodies, and enzymes tailored to meet an infant's needs.*
- *Most infants are ready to transition to solid foods around six months of age. Starting with iron-rich options like fortified cereals and pureed meats supports brain development, while gradually introducing other foods helps expand an infant's palate and reduce allergy risks.*

Developmental Milestones

The first two years of life represent an extraordinary period of growth and transformation. Infants transition from helpless newborns to active toddlers with unique personalities, mobility, and the beginnings of independence. This stage lays the foundation for future cognitive, physical, and emotional development, making it critical for parents to understand what to expect and how to support their child's progress. While many milestones apply universally, subtle differences can offer insights into their developmental trajectories, particularly in girls.

Cognitive milestones in the first two years focus on the infant's ability to process information, learn from experiences, and interact with their environment.

During this time, a child's brain grows astonishingly, forming connections that support memory, problem-solving, and communication.

Birth to 6 Months: Newborns are primarily driven by reflexes but quickly begin recognizing faces, especially their mother's, within the first few weeks. By three months, most infants can track moving objects and respond to familiar voices, indicating early memory formation. Girls may show a slight advantage in visual recognition tasks, likely due to their faster maturation of specific brain regions involved in processing social cues.

6 to 12 Months: Object permanence, the understanding that objects continue to exist even when out of sight, typically emerges around eight months. This concept is critical for memory and problem-solving. Girls often excel in early communicative behaviors, such as pointing, clapping, and imitating words, reflecting their advanced language development at this stage.

12 to 24 Months: By their first birthday, many children can respond to simple commands, recognize familiar objects by name, and use basic problem-solving skills. By two years, toddlers begin combining words to form short sentences and may engage in symbolic play, such as pretending to feed a doll or mimic adult activities. Girls are often more advanced in vocabulary acquisition and imaginative play than boys.

Parents should consult a pediatrician if their child shows difficulties with focus, limited eye contact, or delayed milestones such as lack of interest in exploring their surroundings or failure to respond to their name by 12 months.

Physical milestones during this period focus on motor skills, which can be divided into two categories: gross motor skills (movement of large muscles) and fine motor skills (control of smaller muscles). Girls and boys generally follow similar patterns, but subtle differences emerge in how these skills are mastered.

Birth to 6 Months: Newborns display reflexive movements, such as grasping and rooting. Most infants can lift their heads while on their tummy by four months, and many begin rolling over by five to six months. Fine motor skills, such as holding objects, emerge during this time. Girls may show greater precision in their hand movements earlier than boys.

6 to 12 Months: Sitting independently and crawling are typical milestones during this stage, with standing and cruising along furniture following shortly after. By nine months, infants develop a pincer grasp, allowing them to pick up small objects. Girls often exhibit more excellent dexterity in tasks requiring hand-eye coordination.

12 to 24 Months: Walking independently is a significant milestone that occurs around the one-year mark. By 18 months, many children can climb stairs with assistance and run with growing confidence. Fine motor skills progress to tasks such as stacking blocks, turning pages in a book, and using a spoon. Girls may excel in these areas due to their earlier development of precision and control.

Concerns arise if a child has difficulty holding their head up by three months, cannot sit by nine months, or cannot walk independently by 18 months. Persistent stiffness or floppiness in muscles also warrants evaluation.

The first two years are vital for **establishing emotional bonds and social awareness**. Infants rely heavily on caregivers for comfort, security, and learning how to navigate relationships. Girls often display heightened sensitivity to emotional cues, an early indicator of their strong social and relational abilities.

Birth to 6 Months: Newborns form attachments through touch, eye contact, and consistent caregiving. By three months, infants begin to smile socially and engage in reciprocal interactions with caregivers. Girls may smile and vocalize earlier, reflecting their social attentiveness.

6 to 12 Months: Separation anxiety and stranger wariness typically appear around eight months as infants become more attached to familiar faces. By the end of this stage, many infants can express a range of emotions, from joy to frustration, and will seek comfort from caregivers when upset.

12 to 24 Months: Toddlers begin to assert independence, often accompanied by temper tantrums. This behavior is typical for emotional development as they learn to navigate autonomy. Girls may display stronger empathy and are usually more responsive to social cues, such as comforting a peer or imitating caregiving behaviors.

Parents should seek guidance if their child shows little interest in social interaction, fails to smile or laugh by six months, or does not engage in basic play behaviors by 12 months.

While all children require love, stimulation, and a nurturing environment, understanding the nuanced needs of girls can enhance their developmental outcomes.

Girls benefit greatly from opportunities to practice verbal communication, engage in imaginative play, and develop fine motor skills through drawing, puzzles, and simple crafts. Emotional support is equally critical, as girls often internalize stress more readily than boys, making early intervention and reassurance essential in fostering their confidence and resilience.

It is important to remember that developmental milestones are general guidelines rather than rigid timelines. Each child develops independently and is influenced by genetics, environment, and unique temperament. While girls may excel in certain areas earlier than boys, fostering a supportive and enriching environment ensures all children can thrive during this critical period of growth.

Did you know?

- *In the first two years of life, infants transition from reflex-driven movements to walking, talking, and engaging in symbolic play, laying the foundation for future cognitive, physical, and emotional development. During this time, girls often excel in language acquisition, fine motor skills, and social cues.*
- *By eight months, most babies develop object permanence, the understanding that objects exist even when out of sight. This milestone supports problem-solving and memory, with girls often showing early advancements in communicative behaviors like pointing and clapping.*

Vaccination and Preventive Health

Vaccination is one of the most effective and vital measures for safeguarding children's health, particularly during the first two years of life. This period represents a critical window in which a child's immune system develops and is most vulnerable to infectious diseases. Girls, like boys, benefit immensely from adhering to recommended vaccination schedules. However, due to biological and cultural factors, it is essential to emphasize specific aspects of preventive health for girls.

Vaccines stimulate a baby's immature immune system to recognize and fight harmful pathogens without causing illness. They protect against life-threatening diseases such as polio, measles, and whooping cough and prevent complications that could lead to chronic health issues or developmental delays.

For girls, vaccination is particularly significant as it can also influence their long-term reproductive health. Certain vaccines, like the rubella vaccine, protect against congenital infections that could impact future pregnancies. Additionally, childhood vaccinations are essential in reducing the spread of diseases in communities, especially in regions where girls may have limited access to healthcare.

Health authorities and national pediatric associations provide comprehensive vaccination schedules to guide parents. Key vaccines for girls in this age group include:

- **Hepatitis B:** Administered shortly after birth, this vaccine protects against liver infection, which could have long-term consequences for girls' health.
- **DTaP (Diphtheria, Tetanus, Pertussis):** This combination vaccine prevents serious bacterial infections that could lead to respiratory distress, muscle paralysis, or death.
- **IPV (Inactivated Polio Vaccine):** Protects against polio that can cause lifelong disability or paralysis.
- **Hib (Haemophilus influenzae type b):** Prevents bacterial meningitis, a condition that disproportionately affects young children and can cause lasting neurological damage.
- **PCV (Pneumococcal Conjugate Vaccine):** Protects against pneumonia and ear infections, conditions that can lead to complications in early childhood.
- **Rotavirus:** Prevents severe diarrhea and dehydration, which are more dangerous in infants and young children.
- **MMR (Measles, Mumps, Rubella):** Administered at 12 months, this vaccine protects against diseases that can cause serious complications, including rubella, which is of particular concern for girls' future reproductive health.
- **Varicella (Chickenpox):** Protects against a common childhood illness that can lead to severe infections or scarring in some cases.

Adherence to the vaccination schedule ensures that girls receive protection at the optimal time when their immune systems can mount the most vigorous defense.

While vaccination protocols do not differ between boys and girls, the health implications of some diseases and their prevention may be particularly important for girls. For example, rubella infection during pregnancy can cause congenital rubella syndrome, leading to severe congenital disabilities. Vaccinating girls ensures immunity, protecting their future pregnancies.

In some communities, girls may face challenges accessing healthcare due to cultural norms or financial limitations. Parents must prioritize equitable access to vaccinations to ensure girls are fully protected.

Parents play a crucial role in ensuring adherence to vaccination schedules. Maintaining accurate immunization records and attending scheduled appointments are critical steps. In addition, educating themselves about vaccine-preventable diseases empowers parents to make informed decisions for their daughters' health.

Vaccination is a medical intervention and a societal commitment to nurturing healthy, thriving children. For girls, this commitment also ensures a foundation for lifelong health and overcoming health inequities that may arise due to social or biological factors. Adhering to preventive health measures during the first two years of life is a gift of protection and resilience, setting the stage for a healthy and fulfilling future.

Preventive health for girls in this age group extends beyond vaccines. Routine check-ups with a pediatrician allow for growth monitoring, early detection of potential health issues, and reinforcement of good hygiene practices. It is also a time to address gender-specific needs, such as proper diaper hygiene to prevent urinary tract infections, which are more common in girls.

Did you know?

- *Vaccination during the first two years of life protects against life-threatening diseases like polio, measles, and rubella.*
- *Preventive health for girls also includes proper diaper hygiene to reduce the risk of urinary tract infections, which are more common in girls, and regular pediatric check-ups to monitor growth and address health concerns early.*

Common Infant Health Issues

The first years of a child's life are marked by rapid development, but they can also be accompanied by health challenges that cause infant discomfort and concern for parents. The most common issues faced during this period are colic, reflux, and teething. While these conditions are generally not life-threatening, they can be distressing for both the baby and the caregivers. Understanding and managing these issues effectively is essential, especially for girls who may experience slight variations in symptoms due to differences in anatomy and temperament.

- **Colic: Unexplained Crying and Discomfort**

Colic refers to episodes of excessive crying in an otherwise healthy infant, typically occurring during the first three months of life. It is often characterized by:

- Intense crying spells, often in the late afternoon or evening.
- Clenched fists, stiffened legs, and an arched back indicate discomfort.
- Difficulty soothing the baby despite feeding, changing, or holding them.

The cause of colic is unknown, but theories include gastrointestinal discomfort, immature digestive systems, or heightened sensitivity to stimuli. Girls are equally likely to experience colic as boys, but some studies suggest they may display slightly different crying patterns, such as more consistent rather than sporadic episodes.

Management Tips for Colic:

- **Soothing Techniques:** Rocking, swaddling, or using white noise can help calm a colicky infant.
- **Dietary Adjustments:** For breastfed babies, mothers may consider eliminating potential irritants like caffeine or dairy from their diet. Hypoallergenic formulas might benefit formula-fed infants.
- **Burping After Feeds:** This helps reduce gas, which may alleviate discomfort.

If crying persists or is accompanied by other symptoms (e.g., fever, vomiting), consult a pediatrician to rule out other conditions.

- **Reflux: Spitting Up and Gastroesophageal Discomfort**

Reflux, or gastroesophageal reflux (GER), occurs when stomach contents flow back into the esophagus, leading to spitting up or mild vomiting. It is common in infants due to immature digestive systems and usually resolves by 12–18 months. Girls may exhibit reflux slightly differently, with less forceful spitting up but more signs of discomfort, such as arching the back or refusing to feed.

Symptoms of Reflux:

- Frequent spitting up after feeding.
- Irritability during or after meals.
- Poor weight gain or signs of feeding aversion in severe cases.

Managing Reflux:

- ❖ **Feeding Adjustments:** Smaller, more frequent feeds can reduce the volume of milk in the stomach, minimizing reflux.
- ❖ **Positioning:** Keeping the baby upright for 20–30 minutes after feeding helps prevent stomach contents from flowing back into the esophagus.
- ❖ **Formula Changes:** For formula-fed infants, thickened feeds or unique anti-reflux formulas may be recommended.

Persistent or severe reflux, known as gastroesophageal reflux disease (GERD), may require medication or further evaluation by a pediatrician.

- **Teething: The First Steps to a Healthy Smile**

Teething begins around 4–6 months, although it can vary widely among infants. For girls, some evidence suggests that teeth may erupt slightly earlier than in boys. This process can cause irritability, discomfort, and disrupted sleep as the first teeth (typically the lower central incisors) break through the gums.

Signs of Teething:

- Increased drooling.
- Desire to chew on objects or fingers.
- Swollen, tender gums.
- Mild irritability and disrupted sleep patterns.
- Occasionally, low-grade fever or loose stools, though these are not direct symptoms of teething.

Tips to Soothe Teething Pain:

- ❖ **Teething Toys:** Provide safe, chilled teething rings or toys for the baby to chew on.
- ❖ **Gum Massage:** Gently rubbing the baby's gums with a clean finger can relieve discomfort.
- ❖ **Cold Compresses:** A cold, damp washcloth can be soothing for swollen gums.
- ❖ **Pain Relief:** For significant discomfort, over-the-counter medications like acetaminophen or ibuprofen (as directed by a pediatrician) can be used.

While colic, reflux, and teething are common and usually self-resolving, sure signs warrant medical evaluation:

- Persistent vomiting or signs of dehydration in cases of reflux.
- Fever, blood in stools, or significant weight loss may indicate an underlying condition.
- Excessive crying or inconsolability that does not improve with typical interventions.

Although these conditions affect both boys and girls, it is essential to consider each child's needs and sensitivities. Girls may exhibit subtler cues of discomfort, making parental attentiveness even more critical. Parents can help their daughters navigate these common early health challenges by providing comfort, reassurance, and appropriate care while fostering a strong foundation for growth and well-being.

Did you know?

- *Colic, marked by excessive crying and discomfort in infants, often peaks during the first three months of life. While the exact cause is unknown, soothing techniques like rocking, swaddling, and dietary adjustments for breastfeeding mothers can help ease a baby's distress.*

- *Teething typically begins around 4–6 months, with girls sometimes experiencing earlier tooth eruptions than boys. Chilled teething toys, gum massages, and cold compresses can help soothe swollen gums and relieve discomfort.*

Health in Early Childhood (2-6 Years)

Early childhood, encompassing the ages of 2 to 6 years, is a transformative period marked by rapid physical growth, cognitive development, and emotional maturation. During this stage, children assert their independence, form social bonds, and develop foundational habits that influence long-term health and well-being. This phase is particularly significant for girls as they often demonstrate early advancements in verbal communication, emotional awareness, and fine motor skills, underscoring the importance of tailored support during these formative years.

Health in early childhood extends beyond physical growth to include nurturing behavioral and emotional **resilience**. Social skills flourish as children learn to navigate friendships, express their feelings, and cope with challenges like tantrums and frustrations. With their heightened sensitivity to emotions and social cues, girls often benefit from guided opportunities to explore these skills through play and early education, which are vital for fostering confidence and empathy.

Sleep also plays a pivotal role in early childhood health.

Establishing consistent routines supports emotional regulation, cognitive functioning, and physical growth.

Girls, who may be more affected by disruptions to their environment, require calm and predictable bedtime practices to ensure quality rest. Addressing common sleep disturbances, such as nightmares or bedtime anxiety, is essential for their overall well-being.

Safety remains a priority as children explore their environments with growing curiosity and energy. Girls, while often showing greater caution compared to boys, still face risks of injuries, including falls, choking hazards, and playground accidents. Proactive safety measures and education about safe behaviors help balance their natural independence with the need for protection.

This chapter focuses on the unique aspects of health during early childhood, emphasizing the importance of nurturing social-emotional development, promoting healthy sleep habits, and preventing injuries. By creating a supportive environment, parents and caregivers can help girls thrive during these critical years, setting the stage for a lifetime of physical and emotional well-being.

Behavioral and Emotional Development

Between the ages of two and six, children undergo significant growth in their behavioral and emotional development, shaping their ability to interact with others, regulate emotions, and explore the world around them. For girls, this period often brings a unique blend of emotional sensitivity, early verbal skills, and a growing desire for connection and affirmation. Understanding these developmental milestones and providing appropriate support is essential for fostering healthy emotional and social growth.

Children begin to navigate social interactions with peers and adults during this stage. Girls may show an early inclination toward cooperative play and empathetic responses, often mimicking behaviors they observe in caregivers or older siblings. This natural tendency toward nurturing and collaboration is an opportunity to reinforce positive social skills.

However, **emotional outbursts** and **tantrums** remain a standard part of early childhood. While girls may verbalize their frustrations more effectively than boys, they are not immune to intense emotional reactions. These episodes often stem from a limited ability to process complex emotions or unmet needs for attention and understanding.

Parents and caregivers can address these challenges by:

- **Validating emotions:** Acknowledging a child's feelings helps them feel understood and supported. For example, saying, "I see that you're upset because you can't play with your toy right now," can soothe and teach emotional recognition.

- **Setting boundaries:** Consistency is critical for helping children learn limits. Girls, who often seek approval, may respond well to calmly delivered explanations about acceptable behaviors.
- **Encouraging self-expression:** Introducing girls to age-appropriate ways of communicating feelings, such as drawing, storytelling, or simple phrases, can reduce frustration and improve emotional regulation.

Play is the foundation of a child's cognitive, emotional, and social development during early childhood. Play often incorporates imaginative scenarios for girls, such as role-playing as caregivers, teachers, or community helpers. These activities enhance their problem-solving skills, creativity, and ability to form relationships. Encouraging diverse play experiences can help girls explore various interests and build confidence in their abilities.

Structured early education programs provide additional opportunities for girls to develop key skills, whether at home or in preschool settings. Girls often excel in verbal communication during this stage, benefitting significantly from activities focusing on language development, storytelling, and group interactions. These programs also promote early academic learning, preparing them for later school years.

Parents can enhance their child's development by prioritizing play and education in the following ways:

- **Facilitating social play:** Arranging playdates or group activities encourages girls to practice sharing, cooperation, and conflict resolution. These experiences lay the groundwork for forming meaningful friendships.
- **Balancing structured and free play:** While girls may enjoy organized activities like dance classes or art workshops, unstructured playtime fosters independence and creativity.
- **Introducing early learning opportunities:** Reading books together, engaging in simple science experiments, or playing educational games can stimulate curiosity and build foundational knowledge.

Early childhood environments benefit girls by nurturing their emotional and social growth while encouraging exploration and resilience. Parents and caregivers can help girls develop the confidence and skills needed to thrive in these formative years by understanding their unique tendencies and providing age-appropriate guidance. The foundation built during this period will support their lifelong journey of self-discovery and growth.

Did you know?

- *Girls between the ages of two and six often show an early inclination toward cooperative play and empathetic behaviors, frequently mimicking caregiving roles observed in adults or older siblings. These activities help foster social skills and emotional intelligence.*
- *Girls typically excel in verbal communication during early childhood, making storytelling, imaginative play, and group interactions particularly effective for developing emotional regulation and building confidence.*

Sleep and Routines

Sleep plays a critical role in the physical, emotional, and cognitive development of children aged 2 to 6. Establishing healthy sleep habits during this period is essential, as it directly impacts a child's ability to regulate emotions, concentrate, and grow. For girls, who often exhibit early sensitivity to social and emotional cues, disrupted sleep can lead to heightened emotional reactivity and difficulty managing daily challenges. Understanding common sleep disturbances and implementing consistent routines can help foster restful sleep and overall well-being.

Several factors can disrupt sleep patterns during early childhood, including developmental changes, environmental factors, and emotional triggers. Girls, who are often more attuned to their surroundings and relationships, may experience sleep disturbances influenced by their heightened emotional awareness.

- **Nightmares and Night Terrors:** Girls may have vivid imaginations, which can contribute to nightmares as they process their daily experiences. Night terrors, although less common, can also occur and are usually characterized by sudden crying or screaming during sleep. While these episodes are unsettling, they typically do not indicate underlying psychological issues and often resolve with age.
- **Separation Anxiety:** Girls may struggle with the concept of independence, leading to difficulty falling asleep alone. This anxiety may manifest as repeated requests for parental reassurance or reluctance to stay in their bed.
- **Changes in Routine:** Even minor disruptions, such as travel, illness, or family stress, can affect sleep patterns. Girls, who often thrive on consistency and predictability, may take longer to adjust to new routines.

Creating a consistent and calming bedtime routine is one of the most effective ways to ensure healthy sleep habits for children. Girls, who often find comfort in structured and nurturing environments, can significantly benefit from routines that provide security and predictability.

❖ **Set a Regular Sleep Schedule:** Establishing a fixed bedtime and wake-up time helps regulate a child's internal clock. Girls may adapt well to this structure, as they often enjoy the sense of order it provides.

❖ **Create a Relaxing Bedtime Routine:** Activities such as reading a story, gently stretching, or listening to calming music can signal a child that it's time to wind down. Girls may enjoy rituals involving storytelling or cuddling, as these activities reinforce emotional bonds.

❖ **Limit Screen Time:** Exposure to screens before bed can interfere with melatonin production, making it harder for children to fall asleep. Encouraging screen-free activities in the hour before bedtime can significantly improve sleep quality.

❖ **Ensure a Comfortable Sleep Environment:** Girls may be more sensitive to environmental factors, such as noise, light, or temperature. A quiet, dimly lit, and cool room can create an ideal setting for restful sleep. Allowing them to choose a favorite blanket or stuffed animal may provide additional comfort.

Even with healthy habits, occasional sleep challenges may arise. Parents and caregivers can support their children through these difficulties by addressing underlying causes and maintaining patience and consistency.

If a girl wakes during the night due to a nightmare or anxiety, providing gentle reassurance without prolonged interaction can help her feel secure while reinforcing the importance of self-soothing.

For girls struggling with separation anxiety, techniques such as sitting by the bed and gradually moving farther away over time can encourage confidence in sleeping alone.

Significant life changes, such as starting preschool or the arrival of a sibling, may temporarily disrupt sleep. Open communication about these events and extra attention during bedtime can ease the transition.

Establishing and maintaining healthy sleep routines during early childhood provides a foundation for emotional resilience, cognitive development, and physical health. For girls, who often seek stability and connection, consistent bedtime practices promote better sleep and strengthen their sense of security and trust in their caregivers. Parents can help their daughters develop habits that support lifelong well-being by addressing sleep challenges with understanding and care.

Did you know?

- *Girls aged 2 to 6, often sensitive to emotional and social cues, may experience sleep disturbances like separation anxiety or nightmares. Establishing a calming bedtime routine with activities such as storytelling or cuddling can help foster a sense of security and improve sleep quality.*
- *Consistent sleep schedules and limiting screen time before bed are especially beneficial for young children. For girls,*

creating a comfortable sleep environment - quiet, dimly lit, and remarkable - further supports restful and uninterrupted sleep.

Preventing Injuries

Safety becomes a top priority in early childhood as children become increasingly mobile, curious, and adventurous. This developmental phase is marked by rapid physical and cognitive growth, sometimes leading to risky situations as young children explore their environment. Girls are often encouraged to engage in more structured play or activities but are not immune to the injuries accompanying this stage of life. While their play may sometimes be less physically intense than boys', it is equally essential to ensure their safety through proactive measures.

During the ages of 2 to 6 years, children develop their motor skills, balance, and coordination, which are still far from fully refined. Girls, often involved in imaginative play or activities requiring fine motor skills, may face specific hazards such as:

- **Choking Hazards**: Girls may play with small toys, beads, or crafting supplies, which can quickly become choking risks if accidentally ingested.
- **Playground Injuries**: While engaging in climbing, running, or swinging, children are susceptible to falls and bumps, particularly when surfaces are not adequately cushioned.
- **Burns and Scalds**: Involvement in pretend play, such as "helping" in the kitchen or playing tea party, can expose girls to hot surfaces, liquids, or utensils.
- **Poisoning**: Brightly colored cleaning products, medications, or even cosmetics can attract children's attention, posing a risk of accidental ingestion.

Proactive Safety Measures

1. **Choking Prevention**

- Ensure all toys are age-appropriate and free from detachable small parts.
- Avoid giving children foods that pose a choking risk, such as whole grapes, hard candies, or large chunks of vegetables.
- Supervise children during meals and playtime to minimize the risk of choking incidents.

2. **Playground Safety**
    - Inspect playground equipment for stability, loose screws, or sharp edges.
    - Encourage children to wear proper footwear and avoid overly loose clothing that could catch on equipment.
    - Choose playgrounds with shock-absorbing surfaces like mulch, rubber, or sand to reduce injury severity during falls.
3. **Burn and Scald Prevention**
    - Teach children about the dangers of hot objects, using clear language to explain what "off-limits" is.
    - Keep hot beverages, pots, and pans out of reach, and turn handles inward when cooking.
    - Use safety locks on ovens, microwaves, and other appliances.
4. **Poison Prevention**
    - Store cleaning supplies, medications, and cosmetics in high, locked cabinets.
    - Educate children about the dangers of consuming unknown substances.
    - Label potentially harmful items with clear warnings and symbols to discourage curiosity.
5. **Falls and Furniture Hazards**
    - Anchor heavy furniture, such as bookshelves and televisions, to prevent tipping accidents.
    - Place barriers on stairs and balconies to restrict access.

- Use non-slip mats in bathrooms and other areas with slippery floors.

Safety measures should not discourage children from exploring their environment or enjoying active play. For girls, who often engage in role-playing or creative games, it's essential to strike a balance between fostering independence and ensuring a secure environment.

Climbing on safe playground equipment or helping with supervised activities at home builds confidence and physical skills. Teach children safety basics, such as looking both ways before crossing the street or asking for help when handling unfamiliar objects. Activities like dance, gymnastics, or crafts entertain and teach coordination and responsibility when guided by adults.

Parents play a crucial role in injury prevention. Close supervision and a proactive approach to eliminating hazards are key to reducing risks. Encourage girls to express any discomfort or fear during play, as their ability to communicate these feelings is essential to keeping them safe. Additionally, teach girls that it is okay to say "no" when they feel unsafe, fostering autonomy and confidence in decision-making.

Careful planning and attentive caregiving can minimize the risk of injuries, allowing girls to thrive and explore their world safely while building the skills and confidence they need for future independence.

Did you know?

- *Girls aged 2 to 6, often engaged in imaginative play and crafts, are at risk for specific hazards such as choking on small objects or burns from pretend cooking activities. Supervision and proactive measures, like securing small toys and keeping hot items out of reach, are essential for their safety.*
- *Teaching safety basics, such as looking both ways before crossing the street and expressing discomfort, helps girls build independence and confidence while exploring their world safely.*

A Few Words About the Structure of the Sexual Organs

When parents bring their newborn home from the maternity hospital and examine it closer, they may realize that distinguishing a girl from a boy without examining the external genitalia is nearly impossible. This observation holds true even though boys generally weigh slightly more at birth. The most significant physical distinction between the sexes lies in the structure of their external and internal genital organs.

Understanding the anatomy and function of the human body is not just academic; it can help prevent many future mistakes, particularly when considering medical interventions. What may seem helpful now can sometimes cause harm if guided by myths or misinformation. Unfortunately, many people only begin learning about their bodies when health problems arise, disrupting their lives. Few children are taught about the structure and function of their bodies beyond hygiene basics. As a result, foundational knowledge about anatomy often remains a mystery, leaving people vulnerable to misconceptions and unnecessary medical procedures.

A common mistake parents make is comparing their children's development and health to adult standards based on their experiences and sensations.

This tendency is especially pronounced among mothers observing their daughters' reproductive anatomy and function. Most women don't remember how their bodies appeared or functioned during early childhood, ages three, five, or seven, or even details from adolescence, such as the appearance of their external genitalia or the presence of vaginal discharge. Young girls typically don't focus on these topics except during natural phases of curiosity about gender differences, which is an essential and healthy part of child development. Unfortunately, parents often respond harshly to such curiosity, unknowingly fostering shame or confusion.

Many women unconsciously compare their daughters' development to their own adult experiences. It may involve assumptions about genital appearance, vaginal discharge, or menstrual cycles.

However, equating a child's physiology with adult norms often leads to unnecessary concerns and, in some cases, over-treatment or medicalization. Over generations, this can create a cycle of "inherited" diagnoses, where a mother's anxieties about her own body are transferred to her daughter.

It is vital to recognize that a mother's past experiences do not necessarily reflect her daughter's development. While hereditary factors certainly play a role and will be explored in later chapters, many concerns arise from misunderstandings about what is normal for a child's developmental stage. These misunderstandings often lead to unwarranted worry over children who are perfectly healthy.

Monitoring a young girl's external genitalia, paying attention to any vaginal discharge, and later tracking menstrual regularity during adolescence are all important. However, these activities must be carried out with sensitivity and respect. A parent's role is not only to protect but also to foster trust and understanding.

Forcing frequent or invasive monitoring or asking probing questions about menstruation can lead to feelings of discomfort, shame, or embarrassment in growing girls. As children mature, they may perceive such monitoring as intrusive, potentially straining the parent-child relationship. Building trust and open communication from the earliest years is far more effective than waiting for issues to arise. When a girl feels safe and understood, she is more likely to share concerns about her body without fear of judgment or embarrassment.

Any approach involving force, aggression, or excessive scrutiny can backfire, creating mistrust and emotional distance. Instead, fostering a relationship based on openness and respect allows parents to guide their daughters effectively while respecting their autonomy.

If parents notice irregularities, avoiding panicking or rushing to the doctor is crucial. While monitoring is essential, situations requiring urgent medical attention are relatively rare. Most concerns can "wait" until calmer, allowing parents to gather their thoughts and seek appropriate guidance without overwhelming their child. Panic often leads to rushed decisions and heightened anxiety, both for the parent and the child.

Suggestions for Parents

1. **Educate Yourself First**: Before addressing your child's health, ensure you have reliable knowledge about anatomy and development. Consult reputable books or healthcare professionals for accurate information.
2. **Avoid Overreacting**: Many minor irregularities are harmless and self-resolving. Observe patterns over time and consult a pediatrician only when truly necessary.
3. **Encourage Open Communication**: Foster an environment where your child feels comfortable discussing their body and health. This foundation of trust can prevent misunderstandings and unnecessary stress as they age.
4. **Respect Boundaries**: Monitor health respectfully without crossing boundaries that could make your child feel embarrassed or violated. Explain why certain checks are necessary in a way they can understand.

Did You Know?

- *The appearance of a young girl's genitalia at birth differs significantly from that of an adult woman. This is due to the influence of maternal hormones during pregnancy, which temporarily alter the size and shape of the external genitalia. These changes naturally resolve in the first weeks or months of life.*

- *Children's bodies follow unique developmental patterns; what may seem unusual in a child is often perfectly normal for their age.*

Is a Gynecological Exam Necessary, and at What Age?

In most countries, if a woman gives birth in a medical facility, the newborn's first examination is conducted by a neonatologist or a pediatrician specializing in newborn and infant health. In complicated pregnancy cases, the mother may consult with a neonatologist even before delivery to discuss developmental concerns, the best approach to delivery, and how potential issues may affect labor and the baby's health.

If the pregnancy is uncomplicated, such consultations are typically unnecessary. After birth, the obstetrician or midwife assesses the baby's condition, including a general physical examination and confirmation of the baby's sex. If a pediatrician is present in the delivery room, they may carry out this initial assessment instead, which includes a brief examination of the external genitalia. For a girl, this initial check could be considered her first "gynecological" exam.

In most countries, a family doctor or pediatrician provides ongoing care for children. These physicians oversee growth, development, and general health, with referrals to specialists like pediatric gynecologists when necessary. However, frequent pediatric gynecologist visits are uncommon and reserved for cases requiring specialized diagnostics or treatment. Adolescent gynecologists are more widely available, focusing on issues like menstrual irregularities, teenage pregnancy, contraception, and other challenges faced by adolescent girls.

Among medical professionals, the consensus is that gynecological exams are only necessary when symptoms or concerns about the reproductive system arise, regardless of age. For a healthy child, the first formal gynecological visit is generally recommended during adolescence, typically between 13 and 15 years of age. This initial visit is often limited to an external examination and a conversation about reproductive health.

A manual gynecological exam is usually recommended at age 21 or earlier if the young woman is sexually active or experiences specific symptoms. These symptoms may include:

- Abundant vaginal discharge with an unpleasant odor or yellow-green, purulent coloration.
- Bloody discharge before the onset of menstruation (common in preschool or early school-aged children).
- Persistent discomfort, lower abdominal pain, or itching or burning associated with vaginal discharge.
- Difficulty or pain with urination.
- Signs of early puberty.
- Absence of menstruation after age 16.
- Heavy or painful menstruation that interferes with daily activities.
- Suspected or confirmed sexual abuse.
- Suspected pregnancy.
- Questions or concerns about contraception.

A parent, guardian, or caregiver is generally required during gynecological exams for minors. This ensures the child feels supported and protected. However, adolescent girls typically have the right to request a private consultation with a doctor.

Key guidelines for ensuring a respectful and supportive environment during exams include:

1. **For children under the age of consent**: A parent or guardian must be present, except in emergencies.
2. **For adolescents (typically 15 and older)**: In many countries, they have the legal right to attend a gynecological exam without a parent or guardian present. This protects the adolescent's privacy, particularly when discussing sensitive issues like sexual activity, contraception, or abuse.

3. **Informed consent**: Regardless of age, the child or adolescent must understand the purpose and process of the exam and obtain consent. Forced exams are not only unethical but often punishable by law.

Gynecological exams can be intimidating, especially for young girls. Many feel heightened anxiety about exams involving intimate areas, and this stress may be exacerbated if they don't understand why the exam is necessary. To alleviate these fears, doctors should follow these principles:

- **Explain the procedure clearly**: The doctor should discuss the exam's purpose and benefits in age-appropriate language.
- **Ensure the child feels safe**: Reassure her that the exam is voluntary and that no one will force her to undergo it against her will.
- **Encourage questions**: Allow the child or parent time to ask questions and clarify doubts.

For young children, examinations of the vagina, uterus, or ovaries may require general anesthesia to minimize discomfort. In such cases, discussing the potential risks and benefits with parents beforehand is critical.

Adolescents (usually 15 or older) often have the legal right to attend a gynecological exam without their parents' presence. It ensures confidentiality and fosters trust between the patient and the healthcare provider. Situations in which confidentiality is crucial include:

- Discussing contraception or sexual activity.
- Concerns about pregnancy or sexually transmitted infections (STIs).
- Seeking information about menstrual health.

These rights, however, vary by country and are subject to local laws. In cases where the adolescent's health or safety is at risk, the doctor may override confidentiality by involving the parents or guardians.

To make the experience more comfortable for the child or adolescent:

1. **If the child wishes, involve the parent or guardian.** Parents can provide physical and emotional support, such as holding the child's hand during the exam.
2. **Reschedule if needed**: If a girl is distressed and refuses the exam, rescheduling for a later date is preferable. Forcing an exam can cause psychological harm.
3. **Avoid sedation unless necessary**: Sedatives or calming medications should only be used in exceptional cases, such as with very young children who cannot remain still.

It is vital for parents, particularly mothers, to recognize that a girl's intimate body parts are deeply personal. Any examination of the genital area should be approached with utmost sensitivity and respect to avoid causing emotional trauma or fostering negative attitudes toward medical care.

Parents often worry about their children's health, but it is essential to differentiate normal developmental variations from genuine concerns requiring medical attention. For instance:

- Vaginal discharge is common in young girls and often harmless unless accompanied by other symptoms like foul odor, redness, or pain.
- Adolescents' irregular menstrual cycles are typically normal during the first few years after menarche (the first period).
- Occasional mild abdominal discomfort may be part of normal growth and hormonal changes.

Being observant and maintaining open communication with the child allows parents to balance care and independence.

Did You Know?

- *A girl's first gynecological exam is typically recommended between 13 and 15 years of age, focusing on external observation and education about reproductive health.*
- *In many countries, adolescent girls have the legal right to attend gynecological exams without a parent present to ensure privacy and confidentiality.*

External Genital Organs

Both girls' and boys' external and internal genitalia undergo significant changes from birth until the completion of puberty. Understanding these developmental phases is essential for parents and caregivers to provide appropriate care, avoid misconceptions, and prevent unnecessary medical interventions. Let's examine the anatomy and development of the female reproductive system by age.

In women, the external genitalia, or **vulva**, include the vaginal vestibule, labia majora and minora, clitoris, pubic area, urethral opening, hymen, Bartholin's glands, and vaginal opening.

- ***Perineum***

Few people think about the number of openings in the perineal area and their layout. Moving from the pubic bone down to the anus (toward the tailbone), a woman has three distinct openings: the **urethra** at the top for urination, the **vaginal opening** below it (through which children are born), and finally, the **anus** for excretion. In addition to these central openings, numerous glandular openings are often too small to see without magnification.

Parents rarely explain which opening is used in childbirth, yet this area between the pubic bone and tailbone (extending laterally) is known as the **perineum.**

It's worth noting that the perineal skin is one of the least sanitary areas of the body due to the accumulation of secretions from the urethra, vagina, and anus. These secretions not only build up but also create a favorable environment for microorganisms, typically intestinal bacteria (from the anus) and skin microorganisms like staphylococci, streptococci, and fungi. Cleaning the perineum by rinsing with warm water at least twice a day (ideally after each act of defecation and urination) is crucial for preventing inflammatory conditions of the external genitalia at any age.

The skin between the vaginal entrance and the anus in young girls is thin, richly vascularized, and thus highly sensitive and prone to injury. Women often notice redness and slight bleeding in this area, particularly after straining during defecation, and may observe a white or yellowish coating. Generally, no treatment is necessary; addressing constipation through proper nutrition and maintaining good hygiene of the external genitalia is usually sufficient.

- ***The Pubic Area***

The soft, fatty mound above the vulva covering the pubic bone is known as the **mons pubis** or **mound of Venus**. This fatty area provides protection; during falls or impacts on the lower abdomen, it reduces the force of potential injuries to internal organs. The amount of fatty tissue in this region varies among prepubescent girls, so not all girls have a prominent fat pad in this area. In adult women, the pubic area's skin is densely populated with hair, which begins to grow during puberty due to an increase in male hormones in the girl's body.

- ***Labia Majora and Labia Minora***

The **labia majora** are two skin folds containing a dense layer of fatty tissue that protects the vaginal entrance. They act as a barrier against microorganisms. In girls, the labia majora are closed, providing more effective protection against microbes and foreign objects. With the start of sexual activity, the labia majora may separate slightly. In young girls, the labia majora are smooth and contain less fatty tissue.

The **labia minora** in young girls often extends outward toward the perineum more than in adult women. Usually, they are separated and do not cover the urethral opening. During puberty, the color of the labia minora may change from pale pink to dark red (burgundy) or brown (often referred to as "chocolate" by women). These colors can vary throughout a woman's life and during specific periods, such as pregnancy.

Adolescence also causes changes in the size of the labia minora, and the appearance of the right and left labia may differ. They may have smooth or frilled edges, be asymmetrical, narrow or wide, shiny or matte, etc. These variations are normal and should not cause concern for either the adolescent or the parents.

- ***The Vestibule of the Vagina***

The entire area between the labia and the vaginal opening is known as the **vestibule of the vagina**. This region is constantly kept moist due to secretions from glands and natural vaginal discharge. Irritation of the skin and mucous membranes in the vestibule, whether from chemicals or mechanical factors (such as friction from tight clothing or underwear), can lead to increased secretions, inflammation, and ulceration.

In young girls, this part of the perineum is highly sensitive and easily reacts to any irritation, including temperature. Overheating, sweating, and the accumulation of secretions can quickly lead to redness and discomfort in the vulva area.

- ***The Hymen***

The hymen, a thin membrane located at the entrance of the vagina, is an integral part of the female reproductive system, composed of vaginal mucosa and typically measuring 0.5–2 mm in thickness. Most commonly crescent-like or ring-shaped, the hymen comes in approximately 20 documented variations, all considered normal. Its primary function is protection, a barrier against infections and foreign substances. Typically, it contains one or more small openings to allow menstrual blood to exit during menstruation. Rarely does a congenital absence of the hymen, known as hymenal aplasia, occur, but this condition is scarce and usually harmless.

Maternal estrogens play a significant role in shaping the hymen's appearance in infants. These hormones make the hymen denser, more elastic, and adorned with numerous folds and protrusions. It is pale pink and may bulge slightly outward, though it sits deeper within the vaginal entrance compared to adult women. This characteristic appearance can persist until about age four.

In infancy, the hymenal opening is typically tiny, around 1-2 mm in diameter, and grows approximately 1 mm yearly as the child matures. Variations in hymenal structure, such as multiple small openings or a thin septum dividing the opening, are common anatomical differences and usually do not affect the child's health. However, healthcare providers should assess for any associated abnormalities, such as a vaginal septum, when structural variations are observed.

By ages six to seven, the hymen becomes thinner, smoother, and more sensitive, making it prone to irritation from tight or rough clothing. This sensitivity may lead to redness or discomfort in the vulva area, often misinterpreted as inflammation by inexperienced parents or healthcare providers.

The hymen is relatively resilient, but it is not immune to damage. This risk exists even in early childhood. For example, some healthcare providers unfamiliar with modern pediatric gynecology might attempt to forcibly separate fused labia minora (a condition known as synechiae) during an examination, potentially causing hymenal injury.

Outdated practices, such as prescribing vaginal suppositories or recommending douching for young girls, should be avoided. These interventions not only risk damaging the hymen but also disregard current medical guidelines that prioritize minimally invasive care.

The hymen has long been associated with myths surrounding virginity, leading to unnecessary anxiety and harmful practices. Variations in hymenal structure, such as small multiple openings, are often misconstrued as abnormalities. Additionally, the idea that a woman's hymen remains intact until sexual intercourse is inaccurate. Activities like intense sports, experimentation, or even specific medical procedures can result in hymenal tears without sexual activity.

Adolescents and young adults often face societal pressure regarding hymenal condition and virginity. Misinformation, such as the belief that repeated "stretching" of the hymen with fingers preserves virginity despite intercourse, perpetuates myths. Such practices can cause tiny tears or eventual rupture, challenging these outdated notions.

Parents and educators can play a critical role in debunking these myths by fostering open, honest discussions about the anatomy and its functions. Clear communication helps normalize the natural variations of the hymen and reduces stigma.

Contemporary medical practices emphasize child-centered care to avoid outdated interventions that risk damaging the hymen. Pediatric gynecologists now prioritize non-invasive methods for assessing and treating conditions affecting the external genitalia. Parents are encouraged to seek specialists with expertise in pediatric gynecology if concerns arise, particularly regarding labial fusion, irritation, or hymenal abnormalities.

Building trust between healthcare providers, parents, and the child is essential. Approaches that involve force, intimidation, or outdated practices are not only unnecessary but can cause long-term emotional distress.

- ***Clitoris***

Just below and behind the anterior commissure of the labia majora is the **clitoris**, a highly sensitive area of the female body associated with sexual arousal. Structurally, the clitoris is similar to the male penis, but it lacks a urethra.

In young girls, before the onset of puberty, the clitoris may appear relatively large compared to other parts of the external genitalia. Additionally, **clitoral enlargement (clitoromegaly)** can sometimes be observed in girls whose mothers were taken progesterone or synthetic analogs during pregnancy. In most cases, this condition requires no treatment and resolves independently within the first months or years of the child's life.

Did You Know?

- *The hymen's structure and appearance naturally vary among individuals and change throughout life.*

- *The clitoris contains twice as many nerve endings as the male penis, making it the most sensitive part of the female body.*

Labial Adhesions in Young Girls: Understanding and Managing a Common Condition

Labial adhesions, or synechiae, are common yet often misunderstood in young girls. These adhesions involve the partial or complete fusion of the labia minora and are generally acquired rather than congenital. While labial adhesions are sometimes misdiagnosed or overtreated, they rarely cause serious health issues and often resolve independently without intervention.

Labial adhesions typically develop between 3 months and 3 years of age, with the highest incidence occurring between 13 and 23 months. They are uncommon in newborns unless associated with congenital anomalies of the external genitalia. Despite being relatively frequent, the true prevalence of labial adhesions is poorly documented, as many healthcare systems do not routinely examine asymptomatic children for this condition.

It is estimated that 2–6% of girls under six may experience labial adhesions. These adhesions are often benign and asymptomatic, requiring no specific treatment. Regular medical check-ups may reveal labial adhesions in otherwise healthy children, but this does not reflect negligence in pediatric care. Instead, it reflects a cautious and evidence-based approach to avoid unnecessary interventions in asymptomatic children.

The primary cause of labial adhesions is local inflammation of the vulvar tissue, often linked to low estrogen levels in young girls. In the newborn period, maternal hormones provide a temporary protective effect, but estrogen levels decline significantly by about three months, coinciding with the potential onset of labial adhesions. Other contributing factors include:

- Inadequate hygiene or improper cleaning practices.
- Fungal infections or bacterial overgrowth.

- Skin irritation from diaper use, harsh soaps, or wet wipes.
- Overheating and excessive sweating lead to local irritation.
- Trauma or micro-tears in the perineal area.

Labial adhesions are often partial and asymptomatic, but in some cases, they can lead to urinary difficulties or increased susceptibility to urinary tract infections (UTIs). Studies suggest that 7% of affected girls may have urinary issues, and about 20% may experience urinary tract inflammation.

Contemporary pediatric guidelines emphasize a non-invasive approach to managing labial adhesions. Most cases do not require treatment, especially if the adhesions are asymptomatic and do not interfere with urination or hygiene. Observational studies indicate that 80% of labial adhesions resolve spontaneously within a year, particularly as estrogen levels rise with age.

Treatment is generally recommended only when labial adhesions cause:

- Urinary retention or significant difficulty with urination.
- Frequent UTIs or chronic inflammation.
- Persistent discomfort or pain.

Treatment Options

1. Observation

No treatment is required in asymptomatic cases. Parents should monitor the condition and ensure proper hygiene, as most adhesions will resolve without medical intervention.

2. Topical Estrogen Creams

Estrogen creams have a 90% success rate and remain a primary treatment option. A typical course lasts 2–6 weeks, though longer courses are unnecessary if separation occurs early. Side effects, such as temporary pigmentation or slight breast enlargement, are rare and reversible.

3. Topical Steroid Creams

Steroid creams are highly effective, with success rates up to 95%. They allow for shorter treatment durations, often requiring no more than three applications.

4. Surgical Separation

Surgical intervention is rarely needed and is reserved for severe cases where adhesions repeatedly reform despite medical treatment or when significant urinary issues persist. Local anesthesia is used to ensure the child's comfort. Post-surgical care often includes topical hormonal creams for 2–4 weeks to promote healing and reduce the risk of recurrence.

Older, invasive approaches to treating labial adhesions, such as manual separation during an office visit without anesthesia, are no longer acceptable. Such procedures can cause pain, trauma, and long-term psychological effects. Additionally, douching or the use of vaginal suppositories in young girls is discouraged in modern pediatric practice, as these interventions risk damaging the hymen and disrupting the natural microbiome.

Recurrence rates for labial adhesions range from 40–50% in girls who continue to wear diapers or experience ongoing vulvar irritation. However, recurrence becomes less common as estrogen levels naturally rise with age. Parents should maintain proper hygiene and monitor for signs of irritation to reduce the likelihood of relapse.

Key Takeaways for Parents

- Labial adhesions are not dangerous: In most cases, the condition is benign and resolves independently with time.
- Observation is often sufficient: No treatment or intervention is needed unless symptoms arise.
- Treatment is minimally invasive: Topical creams are highly effective, while surgical options are rarely necessary and only used in severe cases.
- Education is essential: Parents should be informed about the condition to prevent unnecessary worry and to advocate for their child's comfort and well-being during medical evaluations.

Did you know?

- *Labial adhesions resolve spontaneously in 80% of cases within a year without any treatment. This natural resolution results from the body's development and rising estrogen levels as the child grows.*
- *Labial adhesions recur more frequently in girls who wear diapers. This is due to increased irritation and moisture in the diaper area, which highlights the importance of proper hygiene and frequent diaper changes.*

Inflammation of the External Genital Organs in Girls

Inflammation of the external genital organs is a frequent concern in girls due to the sensitivity of the perineal area and vulva, which are often exposed to sweat, urine, stool, and vaginal discharge. This area's condition can frequently reflect the presence of infections or recent illnesses. Common ailments such as colds, diarrhea, or urinary tract infections (UTIs) may manifest with redness in the external genitalia and increased discharge. This condition is often called nonspecific vulvovaginitis, a topic that will be covered in a separate chapter.

When evaluating inflammation in the perineal area, doctors typically consider several questions to identify potential causes:

- **Does the girl use diapers or a potty/toilet?**

Diaper use is associated with a higher likelihood of inflammation due to prolonged exposure to moisture and irritants.

- **How often and with what products are hygiene routines maintained?**

Using scented soaps, foams, dyes, body washes, or abrasive washcloths can irritate the delicate skin in the vulva area.

- **Is the child's diet balanced, and how regular are bowel movements and urination?**

Changes in the bladder or intestines can lead to skin changes in the perineum.

- **Does the child tend to overheat or sweat excessively?**

Overheating and sweating can create an environment conducive to irritation and infection.

- **Does the child have any parasitic infections, such as pinworms?**

These can cause itching and lead to secondary irritation or inflammation.

- **What illnesses has the child had in the past two months, and what medications were used?**

Recent infections or medications might contribute to changes in the vulvar and perineal area.

These factors are critical when assessing redness or irritation, which may stem from infections, trauma, chemical irritants, friction, or allergic reactions.

Common Causes of Perineal Redness

Fungal Infections (Candidiasis/Thrush):

The most common cause of perineal redness in young girls, mainly if diaper rash has been ruled out, is a fungal infection. Fungi, such as Candida species, are natural inhabitants of the body and colonize newborns from birth. While generally harmless, warm, moist environments, like those created by soiled diapers, promote fungal overgrowth. Symptoms often include redness, ulcerations, white patches, itching, and pain.

- **Treatment:** Antifungal creams are typically effective, but frequent diaper changes and encouraging potty use help reduce prolonged exposure to moisture.

Urinary Tract Infections (UTIs):

UTIs frequently cause painful urination, redness, and vaginal discharge with a strong odor. Girls are more prone to UTIs than boys due to their shorter urethra, which allows bacteria to travel to the bladder more easily. Approximately 10% of girls experience a UTI before adolescence.

- **Common Cause:** Most UTIs in girls are caused by *E. coli*, a bacterium found in the intestines and perineal skin. Congenital abnormalities in the urinary system can also increase the risk of recurrent infections.

Parasitic Infections:

Pinworms commonly cause perineal itching in young children, particularly at night. It leads to involuntary scratching of the anal and perineal areas, which may result in secondary bacterial or fungal infections. While pinworms are not harmful, the discomfort and subsequent scratching can exacerbate symptoms.

Other Causes of Redness and Irritation

While fungal infections, UTIs, and pinworms are among the most common causes, other factors may also contribute to redness in the perineal area, including:

- **Allergic Reactions:** Fragrances in soaps, detergents, or fabric softeners can irritate the sensitive skin of the vulva and perineum.
- **Friction or Trauma:** Tight clothing, synthetic fabrics, or improper wiping can cause irritation or minor injuries.
- **Chemical Irritants:** Overusing hygiene products like bubble baths or perfumed cleansers may disrupt the natural balance of the vulva's microbiota.
- **Dietary Factors:** Diets high in sugar or processed foods can contribute to yeast overgrowth, while constipation can lead to straining and perineal redness.

Although most cases of redness and irritation in the perineum can be resolved with proper hygiene, certain situations require medical intervention. Seek professional care if:

- Symptoms persist despite improved hygiene practices.

- Redness or irritation worsens, or the child develops pain, swelling, or ulcerations.
- There is a noticeable discharge with a foul odor or unusual coloration.
- Recurrent infections or unexplained symptoms appear.

A healthcare provider can help identify the root cause and recommend appropriate treatment to ensure the child's comfort and well-being.

Parent Tips: Creating a Hygiene Routine

Establishing a daily hygiene routine can prevent many common causes of perineal redness. Here are some tips for parents:

1. **Teach Proper Wiping Techniques:** Encourage front-to-back wiping to minimize bacterial spread from the anus to the urethra and vulva.
2. **Choose Hypoallergenic Products:** Opt for fragrance-free soaps and detergents to reduce the risk of irritation or allergic reactions.
3. **Encourage Potty Training:** Transitioning from diapers to the potty can reduce prolonged exposure to moisture and irritants.
4. **Keep the area Dry:** After baths or diaper changes, gently pat the perineal area dry instead of rubbing.
5. **Monitor Clothing Choices:** Ensure children wear breathable, loose-fitting clothing from natural cotton fabrics.

Did You Know?

- *About 10% of girls experience a urinary tract infection before adolescence due to their shorter urethra, which facilitates bacterial migration.*
- *While harmless, pinworms can cause significant discomfort and secondary infections through scratching. They're most active at night, often disrupting sleep.*

Internal Genital Organs

The term "internal reproductive organs" refers to the components of the female reproductive system located inside the body, rendering them inaccessible for direct observation by parents or the girls themselves. It is important to emphasize that under no circumstances should mothers or caregivers attempt to examine or "peek" inside their daughters' vaginas. Such actions not only violate personal boundaries but could also cause harm to the hymen, vaginal opening, or perineum, mainly when done without proper knowledge or medical necessity.

The internal reproductive organs include the vagina, uterus, fallopian tubes, and ovaries. The ovaries are unique as the only hormonal organs within the female reproductive system, even during childhood. In girls, the ovaries remain primarily inactive as reproductive organs until puberty, although they produce minimal hormones before this developmental stage. This hormonal activity is foundational in preparing the body for future reproductive functions.

- ***Vagina***

The vagina is a tubular muscular organ that plays a pivotal role in reproduction and childbirth. During fertilization, it activates sperm, facilitating sperm movement toward the egg. It becomes a part of the birth canal in childbirth, enabling the baby's passage.

The inner surface of the vagina is lined with a mucous membrane characterized by numerous folds, giving it a corrugated, tube-like appearance. This folding provides elasticity, allowing the vagina to accommodate changes during sexual activity and childbirth. Over time, particularly after childbirth, these folds naturally diminish due to stretching and aging.

Unlike other parts of the female reproductive system, the vagina does not have its glands. Vaginal secretions are composed of:

- **Blood plasma** seeps from nearby blood vessels.
- **Cervical mucus**, secreted by the cervix.

- **Shed epithelial cells**, which slough off from the vaginal lining.
- **Microbiota**, primarily bacteria that maintain vaginal health.

In young girls, the vaginal environment is dominated by intestinal bacteria, resulting in secretions that are often yellowish or yellow-green and may have an unpleasant odor. It is usual for prepubescent girls and reflects the unique microbial composition of their vaginal flora at this stage. With puberty, the vaginal microflora undergoes significant changes as lactobacilli become predominant. These beneficial bacteria produce lactic acid, lowering the vaginal pH to create a protective, acidic environment that helps prevent infections.

- ***Uterus***

A girl's uterus undergoes remarkable developmental changes from birth, reflecting its vital role in reproduction. This muscular organ's primary function is to nurture and carry a baby during pregnancy. Menstrual bleeding, a hallmark of reproductive maturity, results from cyclic changes in the uterus's innermost layer, the endometrium. Although the uterus does not produce hormones, its tissues are highly responsive to sex hormones like estrogen and progesterone.

The uterus consists of two main parts:

- **The Cervix**: This lower portion connects the uterus to the vagina through the cervical canal. Its mucosal lining resembles the endometrium and plays a crucial role in reproductive health by producing mucus. However, when ovarian hormone levels increase, cervical mucus production begins only during puberty.
- **The Body**: This more significant upper portion houses the endometrium and is primarily responsible for carrying a pregnancy.

Developmental Changes in the Uterus

1. **Newborn Period**:

- At birth, the cervix is larger than the uterine body, with a 1:2 ratio.
- The uterus measures approximately 3.5 cm in length and 1.4 cm in thickness.
- The endometrium is very thin, and a small amount of fluid in the uterine cavity, often seen during ultrasound, is normal and does not require medical intervention.

2. **Before Puberty**:
    - The uterus is cylindrical, unlike the pear-shaped structure typical in adult women.
    - The cervix and body are roughly equal in size, with a 1:1 ratio.
    - The uterus measures 2.5–4 cm long and is no more than 1 cm thick.
    - The uterus begins to grow between ages 6 and 9; during this stage, the cervix may temporarily become thicker than the body.
3. **Adolescence**:
    - The uterus assumes its characteristic pear shape as the body grows larger than the cervix.
    - The body-to-cervix ratio shifts to 2:1 or 3:1.
    - Dimensions increase to 5–8 cm in length, 3 cm in width, and 1.5–3 cm in thickness.
    - With the onset of menstruation, the thickness and condition of the endometrium vary throughout the menstrual cycle.

Orientation of the Uterus

- Before Puberty: The uterus tilts toward the spine, a position known as a retroverted uterus.
- After Pregnancy and Childbirth: The uterus typically shifts forward, tilting toward the pubic bone.

These changes in size, shape, and orientation reflect the uterus's adaptation to different stages of life, from infancy to reproductive maturity and beyond.

- ***Ovaries***

The ovaries are paired organs that serve two critical functions: producing gametes (egg cells) for reproduction and secreting hormones that regulate the normal functioning of the female body. Nature has designed the ovaries with a remarkable redundancy, such that if one ovary is removed or non-functional, the other can often compensate fully. This ensures the reproductive system continues functioning without significantly impacting fertility or overall health.

Developmental Changes in Ovaries by Age

1. **Newborn Period**:
    - The ovarian volume is approximately one cubic centimeter or slightly more at birth.
    - By the end of the first year, this volume begins to decrease to around 0.67 cubic centimeters and generally remains below one cubic centimeter until age six.
2. **Ages 6–10**:
    - Starting at age six, the ovarian volume gradually increases, reaching an average of 1.2 to 2.3 cubic centimeters (approximately two cubic centimeters) by age ten.
    - Due to their small size and limited blood flow, the ovaries may still be undetectable on ultrasound at this stage.
3. **Early Puberty**:
    - With the rise of pituitary hormones (e.g., follicle-stimulating and luteinizing hormones), ovarian volume increases to around four cubic centimeters.
    - Blood flow to the uterus and ovaries also increases during this time.
4. **Adolescence**:
    - Adolescent girls' ovarian volume averages eight cubic centimeters, but typical values range widely from 2.5 to 20 cubic centimeters. This variability

should be carefully considered before drawing diagnostic conclusions.

The ovary's fundamental structural unit is the **follicle**, which contains a **primary gamete** (egg cell) surrounded by follicular fluid rich in **progesterone**. Follicles mature in preparation for ovulation, a process that begins during puberty.

Prepubescent Girls:

- Detecting follicles via ultrasound in girls under 12 is often challenging due to the lack of well-defined ultrasound standards for ovarian characteristics across different ages. Normal findings may include up to six follicles measuring 4 millimeters or less in each ovary.

Puberty and Adolescence:

- Larger follicles may appear around ages 8–9 as the ovaries become hormonally active. By adolescence, multiple growing follicles may be observed during ultrasound imaging, reflecting the irregular hormonal cycles typical of this stage.

Parents often turn to online resources for explanations after receiving ultrasound results, particularly regarding the number and size of follicles observed in their daughter's ovaries.

Normal Follicular Findings:

Follicles up to 7 millimeters in size are typically considered normal in girls under 12. Larger follicles or an increased number of follicles may emerge during early puberty, signaling the onset of ovarian activity.

Misdiagnosis of Polycystic Ovary Syndrome (PCOS):

During puberty, multiple growing follicles on an ultrasound may resemble **PCOS**, mainly if the ovaries are larger than average. However, in most cases, ovarian size remains more minor than what is typical for PCOS, and these findings reflect hormonal fluctuations and irregular ovulation common in adolescents.

Anovulation (absence of ovulation) is expected during this stage and will be discussed in more detail in another chapter.

The Mystery of Nature Every Woman Should Know

As we explore the changes in girls' ovaries during puberty and the development of menstrual cycles, it becomes crucial to understand what happens in the ovaries during different phases of life. This knowledge is essential for grasping how a girl's reproductive health, and that of a future mother, is shaped from her time in the womb through her early twenties.

The ovaries contain follicles, each housing a primary egg cell or oocyte. These egg cells begin a series of divisions during fetal development but pause their growth for about 15 years, resuming only with the onset of puberty. This follicle growth and maturation process, known as **folliculogenesis**, is a fundamental aspect of female reproductive biology. Nearly all follicles start as primordial, tiny, dormant structures measuring just 0.03–0.05 mm, invisible to the naked eye. Activating these follicles is a complex and tightly regulated process that begins with puberty, triggering irreversible growth and maturation.

However, an extraordinary and lesser-known phenomenon occurs in the female body: **the massive loss of egg cells throughout specific stages of life**. Despite its importance, this process is rarely discussed, even though it profoundly impacts a woman's reproductive potential. Once the reproductive organs are formed during embryogenesis, the female body undergoes significant oocyte depletion, the reasons for which remain largely mysterious. While hormonal fluctuations play a key role in follicle maturation, primordial follicles are unaffected by sex or pituitary hormones, suggesting that other mechanisms drive their loss.

There are three critical periods when this loss of germ cells accelerates dramatically. The **first** occurs during the fetal stage, around 20 weeks of gestation, when a female fetus's ovaries contain approximately 6–7 million germ cells. During this time, follicles begin to form. Following an initial division, the egg cells enter a dormant state until adolescence. Despite their dormancy, the number of oocytes continues to decline from this point forward. Notably, many follicles never mature or yield viable eggs, as only a fraction of these cells will complete their development during a woman's reproductive years.

The **second** period of rapid depletion happens during the first year of life, leaving a young girl with only 300,000–500,000 oocytes. By birth, this number drops to 1–2 million, losing nearly 80% of the original supply. This stage coincides with a unique hormonal environment, as the infant's body still retains high levels of estrogen and other hormones from the placenta. During this time, some follicles begin to grow. However, as placental hormones rapidly diminish and the newborn's estrogen levels remain very low, many follicles fail to mature and degenerate. This phase marks a significant reduction in the ovarian reserve.

The ovaries are hormonally inactive before puberty. With the onset of puberty, oocyte maturation begins, setting the stage for ovulation. This process is accompanied by dynamic changes in the structure of reproductive cells and significant shifts in the fluid composition and volume within the follicles.

The **third** significant reduction of eggs occurs at puberty. When a girl experiences her first menstrual period, her ovarian reserve is reduced to approximately 300,000–400,000 eggs. As estrogen levels rise during puberty, many follicles begin to grow. However, most of these follicles will not reach maturity and will regress.

By the end of puberty, the number of oocytes declines further, leaving about 25,000 in each ovary. This gradual reduction continues throughout a woman's life.

After puberty, as menstrual cycles stabilize, the ovaries continue their dynamic process of follicular development. Approximately 70 follicles begin to grow each month, though typically only one reaches ovulation, and even this does not always occur. **The maturation of a follicle is a gradual process, requiring up to 180 days.** This means a woman loses about 70 follicles or more every month, regardless of whether ovulation happens.

Any surgical procedure involving the ovaries or pelvic organs can lead to the loss of ovarian reserve, reducing a woman's finite number of egg cells. Such interventions require careful consideration to avoid unnecessary depletion of this reserve.

Most women enter a phase of accelerated oocyte loss around the age of 37. When the number of remaining oocytes in the ovaries drops to approximately 1,000, menopause begins. For most women, this transition occurs around 50, marking the end of natural fertility.

A woman's ovaries are dynamic organs that constantly change her life. The germ cells within the ovaries mature into egg cells and play a vital role in producing female sex hormones, male sex hormones, and progesterone. These cells are non-renewable and cannot be regenerated once lost. No treatments or methods are available to preserve or replenish the ovarian reserve.

For parents envisioning their daughters as future mothers, it is crucial to prioritize the protection of their ovarian health. Avoiding unnecessary medical or surgical interventions and providing accurate education about reproductive health can empower young women to make informed decisions about their bodies and fertility.

Did You Know?

- *The uterus in newborn girls is proportionally smaller than in adults, with the cervix being twice the size of the uterine body. This unique proportion gradually shifts as girls grow, with the uterus taking on its characteristic pear shape during puberty.*
- *A girl is born with about 1–2 million egg cells, but by the time she reaches puberty, only about 400,000 remain. Most of these will never mature, as only 400 eggs are ovulated during a woman's reproductive years.*

Vulvovaginitis

Previously, I mentioned inflammatory processes affecting the external genitalia and the common causes of redness around the vulva and perineal skin. Inflammation of the vulva is known as **vulvitis**, but since the vaginal area is often involved, the term **vulvovaginitis** is typically used. Vulvovaginitis is frequently accompanied by increased vaginal discharge, which is usually yellow or yellow-green and often alarms parents.

It's essential to understand that, until menstruation begins, the vaginal flora in young girls differs significantly from that of adult women. In young girls, the vaginal ecosystem is dominated by intestinal bacteria and lacks the lactobacilli found in adults, which help maintain an acidic pH by producing lactic acid. Various factors can disrupt this balance, leading to the overgrowth of intestinal bacteria or fungi and inflammation. This condition is referred to as nonspecific vulvovaginitis, indicating that the inflammation is caused by microorganisms already present in the vagina and perineal skin, such as E. coli, enterococci, streptococci, or Candida.

Nonspecific vulvovaginitis can also result from non-infectious factors, such as:

- **Friction** from tight or rough clothing.
- **Trauma** to the perineal area often goes unnoticed.
- **Chemical irritants**, including scented soaps, bubble baths, or certain detergents.
- **Improper hygiene practices**, whether inadequate or excessive.

When inflammation is caused by sexually transmitted bacteria, viruses, or parasites, the condition is classified as specific vulvovaginitis. Examples include infections like gonorrhea, chlamydia, or trichomoniasis, which in children raise concerns of sexual abuse and require immediate evaluation and intervention.

The vagina's anatomy makes it particularly vulnerable to such issues. It is situated between the gastrointestinal tract and the urinary system, with only a thin layer of connective and fatty tissue separating these organs. This proximity and shared blood vessels and lymphatic pathways allow bacteria, fungi, or viruses to migrate between these systems under certain conditions.

The large intestine harbors billions of bacteria and fungi necessary for digestion, while the lower urinary tract is often exposed to microorganisms from the perineal skin. Despite frequent urine flushing, some organisms may colonize the urethra and bladder. Under normal conditions, a delicate balance exists between these microbial communities, preventing harm to the pelvic organs. However, illnesses in one system, such as a urinary tract infection or gastrointestinal disturbance, can upset this balance, resulting in inflammation that often affects the vaginal area as well.

The exact frequency of vulvovaginitis in young girls is difficult to determine, as many cases resolve naturally with proper external genital hygiene and never reach a healthcare provider. Among girls who do visit a doctor with relevant symptoms, approximately half are diagnosed with vulvovaginitis. As girls age, embarrassment or fear may prevent them from reporting symptoms to a parent or physician, leading to underdiagnosis in older children.

Studies suggest that 30-60% of vulvovaginitis cases in girls are associated with concurrent urinary tract infections (UTIs), which occur five times more frequently in girls than boys. Determining whether vulvovaginitis or UTI is the primary condition can be challenging. However, treating vulvovaginitis alone resolves related symptoms in approximately 60% of cases.

As noted in the chapter on inflammatory conditions of the external genitalia, numerous factors can lead to redness and inflammation of the vulva. A common cause of vulvovaginitis in girls is an infection from another part of the body, such as the throat, nose, or ears. Infections associated with colds or fevers frequently result in vulvovaginitis, with β-hemolytic streptococcus group A being a common culprit. This bacterium is thought to be transmitted to the perineal area through hand contact, as children often touch their mouths or noses and then handle their genital area, particularly after urination or bowel movements.

Streptococcal vulvovaginitis accounts for approximately 20% of all cases.

While pinworms are a well-known cause of vulvovaginitis in children, other parasitic infections can also lead to this condition. Ascariasis, a parasitic disease caused by roundworms, is common among children and is often identified incidentally during stool examinations. Although ascariasis rarely causes significant harm, its symptoms warrant attention and appropriate management, particularly in the perineal area.

Vulvovaginitis can develop not only due to infections or irritants but also in association with existing skin or systemic conditions, such as atopic dermatitis, psoriasis, or immune system disorders. These factors should be carefully considered during diagnosis to determine the underlying cause and appropriate management.

The most common symptoms of vulvovaginitis include:

- Abundant vaginal discharge, often accompanied by an unpleasant odor (although normal vaginal discharge in girls may also have a mild odor).
- Redness, burning, and itching of the vulva.
- Discomfort or pain during urination.
- General signs of irritation or inflammation around the vulvar area.

In most cases, nonspecific vulvovaginitis does not require medical treatment and resolves independently within a few days if proper hygiene practices are followed. To promote healing and prevent further irritation, consider the following:

- Avoid frequent washing and excessive wiping of the perineal area, especially with dry towels or wet wipes.
- Avoid using scented soaps, bubble baths, or products containing dyes and fragrances that can irritate sensitive skin.
- Change underwear daily, and for younger girls, replace diapers frequently to reduce moisture and discharge buildup.

- Prefer showers over baths if there is heavy vaginal discharge, as baths can increase irritation.

More detailed information on proper hygiene practices is provided in the relevant chapter on perineal care.

Proper bowel and bladder habits are critical for preventing and managing vulvovaginitis:

- Encourage a well-balanced diet rich in fiber and hydration for constipation or diarrhea to support healthy bowel function.
- Teach girls to empty their bladder regularly, ideally every 2–4 hours, to avoid prolonged contact between urine and the perineal skin, which can contribute to irritation.

If vulvovaginitis causes significant discomfort, persists despite adherence to hygiene measures for several days, or if the child's condition worsens (e.g., increased redness, pain, or discharge), it is essential to seek professional medical advice. A healthcare provider can identify the condition's root cause, rule out more serious underlying issues, and recommend appropriate treatment.

Did You Know?

- *Vulvovaginitis in young girls is often caused by non-infectious factors like friction or improper hygiene, and most cases resolve naturally with proper care.*
- *Approximately 20% of vulvovaginitis cases in children are linked to β-hemolytic streptococcus group A, often transmitted through hand contact.*

Health in Middle Childhood (6-12 Years)

Middle childhood, aged 6 to 12, represents a pivotal phase in a child's development. This period bridges the gap between early childhood and adolescence and is marked by remarkable physical, cognitive, emotional, and social growth. During these years, children establish independence, expand their social networks, and build habits that often carry into adulthood.

For girls, this stage is particularly significant as it sets the foundation for the physical and emotional changes of puberty. While boys and girls share many developmental milestones, girls often experience early signs of pubertal changes, such as the growth of breast buds or the appearance of fine pubic hair, toward the end of this phase. These subtle changes can influence how girls perceive their bodies and self-esteem, making this an opportune time to nurture positive body image and confidence.

The school years also bring heightened exposure to new environments, ideas, and social pressures. Friendships become more profound and more complex, and academic demands increase. This stage is often accompanied by a surge in curiosity and the desire to master new skills, from learning to play an instrument to excelling in sports or creative arts. Encouraging these pursuits fosters cognitive growth and builds resilience and self-discipline.

Health in middle childhood is multifaceted, encompassing more than physical well-being. Adequate nutrition, regular physical activity, and sufficient sleep are vital for sustaining this age's rapid growth and energy needs. Preventive health measures, such as regular medical check-ups, vaccinations, and dental care, protect children from preventable illnesses. Furthermore, fostering emotional intelligence and teaching effective coping strategies help children navigate the challenges of this stage with confidence.

Discussions about health and hygiene become increasingly crucial for girls as they begin to encounter early signs of puberty. Open communication about these changes, supported by accurate and age-appropriate information, can ease the transition and promote a sense of normalcy.

Middle childhood is also a critical time to instill lifelong habits of safety and self-care. Whether teaching road safety, ensuring proper use of technology, or encouraging responsible decision-making, these lessons equip children to handle the increasing independence that comes with this stage.

As caregivers and educators, we guide and support children during this formative time, creating a solid foundation for their journey into adolescence. By addressing the unique needs of girls and recognizing the importance of holistic health, we can ensure that they emerge from middle childhood healthy, confident, and ready to embrace the future.

Physical Activity and Fitness

The middle childhood years, from 6 to 12, are critical for developing healthy physical activity and fitness habits. This stage presents a unique opportunity for girls to establish a positive relationship with their bodies and movement, setting the foundation for lifelong health and confidence. While societal norms often emphasize girls' physical activity less than boys', it is vital to encourage girls to engage in active play and sports. These activities are essential for physical health and significantly improve emotional well-being, self-esteem, and social skills.

Girls in this age range benefit from various physical activities, from structured sports to unstructured play. Active play, such as jumping rope, climbing, or participating in games like tag, allows girls to explore their abilities in a fun, low-pressure environment. Team sports, such as soccer, basketball, or gymnastics, foster teamwork, discipline, and resilience, while individual activities like swimming, dance, or martial arts help girls develop focus and self-reliance.

Engaging in sports and active play helps girls build:

- **Muscle strength and coordination:** Running, climbing, or balancing activities strengthen muscles and improve motor skills.

- **Bone health:** Weight-bearing exercises, such as jumping or skipping, are essential for girls as they lay the groundwork for preventing osteoporosis later in life.
- **Emotional resilience:** Sports and physical play provide a constructive outlet for stress and teach valuable lessons in perseverance and dealing with challenges.

Addressing cultural stereotypes that may discourage girls from participating in physical activities is crucial. Parents, educators, and coaches should create supportive environments emphasizing effort and enjoyment over competition. Encouragement from role models, whether parents, teachers, or female athletes, can inspire girls to explore activities they may not have considered.

With the increasing prevalence of screens in everyday life, sedentary behaviors pose a significant challenge to children's physical health, especially for girls, who may be more inclined toward quiet, indoor activities. Excessive screen time, whether watching television, using tablets, or engaging in social media, can lead to a sedentary lifestyle, which negatively impacts physical health, disrupts sleep patterns and contributes to weight gain.

To counteract these effects, **set boundaries for screen time.** Clear limits, such as no more than one to two hours of recreational screen use per day, help children develop a balanced approach to technology. **Encouraging alternative activities** like arts and crafts, reading, or outdoor play ensures that screens are not the default source of entertainment. Parents who engage in regular physical activity set an example for their children. Family activities like hiking, biking, or walking can make exercise enjoyable and inclusive.

Girls often face unique challenges in adopting an active lifestyle, including societal pressures and body image concerns that may arise as they approach puberty. Physical activity can serve as a powerful tool for combating these issues. Activities that girls find enjoyable and rewarding can enhance self-confidence and promote a positive body image. For instance, a girl who enjoys dance classes may develop a strong sense of body awareness and grace, while another who excels in soccer may gain confidence in her abilities and teamwork skills.

Schools, communities, and families are critical in promoting fitness among girls. Schools should prioritize physical education programs that include activities appealing to diverse interests. Communities can offer accessible sports leagues and recreational programs designed to be welcoming and inclusive for girls of all skill levels. Families, meanwhile, can encourage physical activity by creating opportunities for movement, such as weekend outings to the park or family fitness challenges.

Physical activity during middle childhood is about more than physical health. It empowers girls to discover their strengths, build confidence, and cultivate a lifelong appreciation for movement. By emphasizing active play and addressing sedentary behaviors, we can help girls thrive physically and emotionally as they navigate this critical stage of development.

Dental and Oral Health

Dental and oral health are fundamental aspects of a child's overall well-being, particularly during middle childhood (6–12 years), when lifelong habits are formed. For girls, this stage often involves a heightened interest in appearance and self-care, making it an opportune time to instill the importance of maintaining a healthy smile. Good oral hygiene not only prevents cavities and gum disease but also plays a role in building self-confidence, especially as children navigate social environments and peer relationships.

Middle childhood is a critical period for oral health as permanent teeth gradually replace baby teeth. Establishing good dental care routines during this time is essential to prevent issues such as cavities, gum disease, and malocclusion, which can have lasting effects on oral and overall health. For girls, who often display an early interest in personal grooming and appearance, this period provides an ideal window to emphasize the significance of a radiant, healthy smile.

Brushing at least twice daily with fluoride toothpaste and flossing daily are non-negotiable elements of good oral hygiene. Proper brushing removes plaque, a sticky film of bacteria that can lead to cavities and gum disease. Flossing helps clean between teeth where a toothbrush cannot reach, preventing decay and gum inflammation. Parents should guide and supervise their children until they master these techniques. For girls, personalized tools, such as toothbrushes in favorite colors or with fun designs, can make these routines more engaging and enjoyable.

Visiting the dentist every six months for cleanings and exams is critical for maintaining oral health. Dental visits not only help prevent cavities but also provide an opportunity for professional advice on proper care and early detection of issues. For girls who may be self-conscious about their appearance, these visits can reinforce the importance of a healthy smile and provide reassurance about aesthetic concerns.

A balanced diet plays a pivotal role in oral health. Foods rich in calcium, such as dairy products, leafy greens, and fortified cereals, strengthen teeth and gums. Limiting sugary snacks and drinks, which contribute to tooth decay, is equally important. Parents can encourage girls to choose healthier options by explaining the connection between good nutrition and a beautiful smile.

In middle childhood, orthodontic issues, such as misaligned teeth or improper bites, become apparent. Early detection and intervention, known as "interceptive orthodontics," can address these problems before they worsen, potentially minimizing the need for extensive treatments later.

Dentists and orthodontists often recommend an evaluation around age 7 to assess jaw alignment, spacing, and bite patterns. Early detection allows timely interventions, such as space maintainers or expanders, to guide the proper alignment of permanent teeth. These evaluations can reassure parents and help children feel proactive about their dental health.

Braces or clear aligners may be introduced to correct misaligned teeth or jaw issues for some children during this stage.

While these treatments can initially seem daunting, emphasizing their long-term benefits, such as a beautiful, functional smile, can help girls feel optimistic about the process. Explaining the aesthetic improvements that come with orthodontic care can particularly motivate girls who are beginning to care more about their appearance.

Creating a fun and supportive environment for dental care can make a significant difference. For girls, who may be more willing to embrace grooming routines, incorporating small rewards, like stickers or progress charts, can motivate consistent practice. Parents can also encourage healthy habits by modeling good oral hygiene and making dental care a family activity.

For many middle-aged girls, self-esteem is closely tied to their appearance and smile. A healthy, clean smile fosters confidence and can help children feel more comfortable interacting with peers and participating in social activities. Addressing dental issues early and reinforcing positive habits can empower girls to take pride in their oral health and appearance.

Parents can lay the foundation for a lifetime of healthy habits and self-assurance by prioritizing dental hygiene and addressing orthodontic needs during middle childhood. Teaching girls the value of oral care promotes physical health and enhances their emotional well-being, preparing them to face the future with confidence and a radiant smile.

Building Healthy Habits

Middle childhood (6–12 years) is crucial for instilling lifelong habits related to nutrition, hygiene, and self-care. This stage is particularly significant for girls as their developing awareness of appearance, health, and personal responsibility shapes their attitudes toward these essential aspects of well-being. Encouraging healthy routines during these years lays a solid foundation for adolescence and beyond.

Proper nutrition is central to a child's growth, energy levels, and overall health. For girls, whose bodies begin preparing for the physical and hormonal changes of puberty during this stage, balanced diets play an even more critical role.

1. **Balanced Meals**

A diet rich in fruits, vegetables, whole grains, lean proteins, and dairy products provides the essential nutrients for bone growth, muscle development, and overall health. Calcium—and vitamin D-rich foods, such as yogurt, milk, and leafy greens, may benefit girls by supporting strong bones and reducing the risk of future osteoporosis.

2. **Healthy Snacking**

Girls often require energy-dense snacks to fuel their active days, so parents should emphasize wholesome options like nuts, fruit, cheese, and whole-grain crackers. These alternatives help maintain steady energy levels without relying on sugary or processed foods, contributing to weight gain and dental issues.

3. **Involvement in Food Choices**

Teaching girls about meal preparation and nutritional labels empowers them to make healthier choices. Encouraging them to participate in grocery shopping or cooking introduces a sense of independence and fosters a positive relationship with food.

Personal hygiene is another cornerstone of health and well-being during middle childhood. For girls, developing a routine for cleanliness not only prevents illness but also supports self-esteem as they become more socially aware.

Girls should be encouraged to wash their hands frequently, bathe regularly, and brush their teeth twice daily. These habits help ward off common infections and ensure they feel confident in their interactions with peers.

Some girls may experience early skin changes, such as increased oiliness or minor blemishes, so gentle skin cleansing routines can help prevent acne. Also, teaching proper hair care, including combing and washing, allows girls to develop self-care skills tailored to their needs.

Allowing girls to select their hygiene products, such as mild soaps, shampoos, and moisturizers, fosters a sense of ownership over their routines. Introducing discussions about the importance of deodorant and other hygiene practices before puberty ensures they are prepared for upcoming changes.

Middle childhood is ideal for teaching **self-care skills** that promote independence and responsibility. Girls often exhibit earlier maturity than boys and are particularly receptive to learning and practicing these skills.

Time Management

- Helping girls establish schedules for homework, playtime, and personal routines teaches them the value of organization and balance. A visual aid, like a daily checklist, can guide them as they navigate their growing responsibilities.

Emotional Self-Care

- Girls should be encouraged to express their emotions and seek support when needed. Journaling or mindfulness exercises can help them manage stress and build emotional resilience.

Positive Body Image

- Middle childhood is a critical time for shaping how girls view their bodies. Reinforcing the idea that health is more important than appearance and celebrating their unique qualities fosters a positive self-image.

By focusing on nutrition, hygiene, and self-care skills, parents can guide girls toward developing habits that support their physical health and nurture their confidence and independence. These foundational practices empower girls to enter adolescence with the tools they need to thrive.

Puberty in Girls

Puberty in girls is a gradual, multifaceted process that unfolds over several years, often beginning well before parents notice visible secondary sexual characteristics. Contrary to popular belief, the foundation of puberty is established long before physical maturity becomes apparent.

The key processes that signal the onset of puberty in girls include:

- **Gonadarche** – the activation of the pituitary gland, leading to increased production of gonadotropins that stimulate the ovaries.
- **Adrenarche** – a rise in androgen levels produced by the adrenal glands, contributing to early changes such as body odor and the growth of fine body hair.
- **Thelarche** – the initial development and growth of breast tissue.
- **Pubarche** – the appearance of pubic hair, often one of the earliest external signs of puberty.
- **Growth spurt** – a rapid increase in height and weight, one of the most noticeable changes during this stage.
- **Menarche** – the onset of the first menstrual period, marking a significant milestone in reproductive maturity.

These terms may seem clinical or complex, but understanding their sequence and significance is crucial for interpreting the natural progression of puberty.

In the 1960s, Dr. Tanner and his colleagues introduced a system for classifying the stages of sexual development in children, now widely known as the Tanner stages. This system evaluates the development of external genitalia, breast tissue, and pubic hair growth in girls, dividing puberty into five stages. Stage 1 represents the absence of visible secondary sexual characteristics, while Stage 5 signifies the completion of puberty.

While the Tanner classification remains a valuable framework for assessing physical signs of puberty, it has limitations. It focuses on visible markers but does not fully account for the internal hormonal and physiological processes that precede these external changes. Many textbooks and medical resources continue to emphasize that puberty begins during adolescence, raising questions about when adolescence itself truly begins.

For many girls, the hormonal precursors of puberty, gonadarche, and adrenarche, may start as early as ages 6–8, long before external signs such as breast development (thelarche) or pubic hair growth (pubarche) appear. This gradual onset underscores the importance of understanding the interplay between visible and invisible aspects of puberty to provide appropriate guidance and support during this critical developmental stage.

Clinical practices often fail to account for these nuances. For example, prescribing hormonal contraceptives to adolescent girls to "regulate" menstrual cycles or treat elevated androgen levels before puberty is complete is a common but misguided approach. Similarly, addressing functional ovarian cysts or other physiological variations in teenagers using outdated principles that equate adolescent physiology with that of adult women can lead to inappropriate interventions. A significant contributing factor is the lack of age-specific reference ranges for hormone levels in diagnostic laboratories, complicating accurate assessments.

The processes of gonadarche (pituitary activation and ovarian stimulation) and adrenarche (increased adrenal androgen production) are closely linked to a third hormonal mechanism: the activation of growth hormones, particularly insulin-like growth factor (IGF). These processes are pivotal in initiating puberty but are often overlooked in standard assessments.

The early phase of puberty, or "pubertal awakening," is characterized by subtle hormonal changes influenced by various external factors beyond genetics.

Nutrition, physical activity, rest cycles, stress levels, socioeconomic conditions, and family dynamics all play a role in determining the timing and progression of puberty. This underscores the complexity of its initiation and highlights the importance of considering these external influences.

Examining the prepubertal phase, the period immediately preceding puberty is crucial to fully understanding adolescence and its associated changes. Recognizing the continuum between these stages allows for a more comprehensive understanding of adolescent development and better support for girls' physical and emotional needs during this transformative period.

Gonadarche

Puberty begins not with the reproductive organs but with the activation of the pituitary gland — a crucial endocrine gland located at the base of the brain in a bony cavity called the *sella turcica*. This gland and its intricate connection to the hypothalamus regulate growth, reproduction, and other vital processes.

The pituitary gland, or hypophysis, comprises an anterior and a posterior lobe. It communicates with the hypothalamus via a sophisticated vascular network between the 10th and 13th weeks of pregnancy. This connection forms the foundation of the **hypothalamic-pituitary-ovarian axis**, which regulates ovarian function. This axis becomes active during puberty and reaches full maturity by ages 21–22. Any unwarranted hormonal interventions during the development of this system can have lasting consequences, including menstrual irregularities and potential infertility.

The anterior pituitary produces multiple hormones that influence various organs, including the ovaries. Since the ovaries are categorized as gonads, the hormones produced by the pituitary that regulate them are called **gonadotropins**. These include:

- **Follicle-Stimulating Hormone (FSH):** Stimulates follicle growth in the ovaries and supports the maturation of egg cells (oocytes).
- **Luteinizing Hormone (LH):** Regulates the corpus luteum after ovulation and influences other ovarian functions.

These hormones also have additional bodily roles, impacting growth and metabolic processes.

The first significant surge of gonadotropin production occurs in girls at around three months of age, following the drop in placental hormones such as progesterone and estrogens acquired in utero. Gonadotropin levels remain elevated in girls for the first one to two years of life (and up to six months in boys), after which they gradually decline. Even so, periodic hormonal fluctuations continue until age four, with a subtle increase observed again.

In adults, gonadotropin production follows a rhythmic, pulsatile pattern. In men, this occurs approximately every two hours, while in women, the rhythm shifts with different phases of the menstrual cycle, occurring every 60–90 minutes. However, in girls, a distinct pulsatile release pattern of gonadotropins does not typically develop until regular menstrual cycles are established, usually by the end of puberty (around ages 19–22).

Around ages 10–11, as some external signs of puberty become evident, the hypothalamus produces **gonadotropin-releasing hormone (GnRH)** during sleep. This triggers an increase in gonadotropins and estrogens, although the balance between luteinizing hormone (LH) and follicle-stimulating hormone (FSH) remains unstable. This initial rise in gonadotropins is insufficient to induce full egg maturation, which is why many menstrual cycles in early adolescence are anovulatory (lacking ovulation). Over time, the synchronization between the hypothalamus, pituitary gland, and ovaries strengthens.

It is essential to understand that the processes of gonadarche (the rise in gonadotropins) and adrenarche (the rise in androgens) are mainly independent. While they occur concurrently during puberty, they are not directly linked. As puberty progresses, gonadotropin production becomes more rhythmic, establishing a pulsatile pattern essential for regulating reproductive hormones like estrogen and progesterone.

This transition from irregular gonadotropin release to a synchronized, pulsatile mode is a defining characteristic of puberty. In girls, this shift is marked by **menarche** (the first menstrual period). In boys, a similar milestone **spermarche** (the first spontaneous ejaculation) occurs, often accompanied by nocturnal emissions, colloquially known as "wet dreams." These milestones signify the culmination of complex hormonal and physiological processes central to human development.

Adrenarche

Adrenarche refers to the increase in male hormone levels in prepubescent and pubescent children, a natural phenomenon often misunderstood or overlooked by parents and healthcare providers. This lack of awareness can lead to unnecessary concern or treatments when elevated male hormone levels are detected in young girls.

The androgen group comprises several hormones, including **dehydroepiandrosterone sulfate (DHEA-S)**, the most abundant androgen in the blood, **dehydroepiandrosterone (DHEA)**, **androstenedione (A)**, **testosterone (T)**, and **dihydrotestosterone (DHT)**. The first three are classified as prohormones or precursors because they can convert into testosterone, indirectly exhibiting androgenic activity. DHT, a metabolite of testosterone, is considered one of its most potent forms.

In children, the initial rise in androgens, primarily DHEA, DHEA-S, and androstenedione, originates in the adrenal cortex. This increase can be detected in laboratory tests as early as age six, though it is more commonly observed around ages seven or eight, marking the start of **adrenarche**.

Elevated androgen levels typically persist throughout puberty. This prolonged presence explains common complaints among adolescents, such as oily skin, acne, and irregular menstrual cycles, which are often typical aspects of physiological development.

There is a widespread misconception that male hormones are inherently detrimental to the female body. Many associate the term "male hormones" with incompatibility with female physiology. However, androgens are integral to many biological processes and serve as precursors to estrogens. Without androgens, the production of estrogens would not be possible. Remarkably, women produce more testosterone and other androgens than estrogen. Although only a tiny fraction of these androgens is converted into estrogens, the amount suffices to support the healthy functioning of the female body.

Androgens, particularly during adrenarche, are not merely hormonal byproducts but play an active role in growth and development. For example, these hormones influence the maturation of the prefrontal cortex and other brain areas, contributing to cognitive development and mental health. Research has increasingly focused on the relationship between hormonal changes and adolescent behavior and mental health fluctuations during this critical stage.

Adrenarche is a phenomenon unique to humans, chimpanzees, and gorillas. It does not occur in most other animal species, underscoring its distinct evolutionary significance. Elevated androgen levels during adrenarche affect various bodily systems, mainly stimulating the development of axillary (underarm) and pubic hair.

While some symptoms associated with androgen increases, such as skin changes or irregular cycles, may seem concerning, they are generally expected and temporary.

Both parents and healthcare providers must understand that adrenarche is a natural developmental stage and does not require medical intervention unless accompanied by significant abnormalities or distress.

Finally, it's essential to recognize the role of progesterone, a steroid hormone that serves as a precursor to adrenal and sex hormones, including androgens and estrogens. Progesterone is not classified as a sex hormone itself but is foundational in the body's hormone synthesis. Supplementing with progesterone, particularly in young girls, can disrupt hormonal balance, depending on the dosage, absorption, and individual health conditions.

By appreciating the intricate interplay of androgens and their broader influence on the body, parents and caregivers can better support the healthy growth and development of adolescents during this transformative stage.

Thelarche and Pubarche

As androgen levels rise around ages 7–8, two closely connected processes typically begin in girls: the development of breast tissue (thelarche) and the appearance of pubic hair (pubarche). These changes represent some of the earliest visible signs of puberty and are significant milestones in a girl's physical development.

Breast budding, or **thelarche**, marks the initial stage of breast development. **Pubarche**, the growth of pubic hair, often occurs in parallel, although the sequence and timing may vary from one individual to another.

Extensive pediatric research has identified several factors influencing the age at which thelarche and pubarche occur. Among the most prominent are genetics, ethnicity, and race. For example, African American girls often begin showing these signs of puberty approximately 1–1.5 years earlier than Caucasian girls.

Early breast or pubic hair development may be observed in girls as young as 4–6 years old. Suppose no other signs of puberty or underlying conditions, such as hormone-related tumors, are present. In that case, these early signs are not typically classified as **precocious puberty** and usually require no medical intervention. Body composition also plays a critical role in pubertal development. In both overweight and underweight girls, breast development may initially go unnoticed due to differences in body fat distribution. Nutrition and physical activity are equally important factors. Girls who participate in intense physical training or sports may experience delayed thelarche due to the impact of rigorous exercise on their hormonal balance and body composition. A separate chapter will explore how sports influence girls' health and development.

It is essential to reassure girls and their parents that breast growth is often not symmetrical. In many cases, one breast may develop faster than the other. This asymmetry is normal and persists into adulthood for many women. If a noticeable size difference between the breasts becomes apparent, explaining that this variation is a natural part of development and does not require intervention is crucial.

In adulthood, some young women may consider cosmetic surgery to address asymmetry. However, such procedures are not recommended during adolescence (under 20–21 years old) when the body is still developing, and hormonal fluctuations can continue to influence breast shape and size.

Parents and caregivers can support girls as they navigate these early stages of puberty by fostering understanding and providing reassurance. This can help build confidence and normalize the changes occurring in their bodies.

In recent decades, girls have experienced puberty at increasingly younger ages compared to previous generations. Breast development, or thelarche, occurs earlier, and the onset of menstruation (menarche) is also advancing.

This trend, often called "acceleration," is frequently attributed to environmental pollution and adverse ecological factors. Over the past 15–20 years, a significant rise in breast reduction surgeries among young women aged 17–22 highlights an increase in breast size during adolescence, further indicating earlier and more pronounced pubertal changes. While environmental factors play a role, they may not fully explain this phenomenon.

Global obesity rates among children and adolescents have also risen sharply, even in developing countries where malnutrition and food insecurity remain concerns. Poor dietary habits, including the consumption of high-calorie, easily digestible foods like refined grains and sugary products, are likely contributing to this trend.

Another under-discussed factor is the use of steroid hormones and other hormonal additives in agriculture, particularly animal farming. These substances are often used to accelerate livestock growth. While regulations exist in many countries to limit hormone levels in food, it's worth noting that food products like chicken or cow's milk a century ago were free from synthetic hormones. This raises questions about their potential role in influencing the earlier onset of puberty.

Growth Spurt

Adolescence is a time when growth rates accelerate significantly in girls and boys, second only to the rapid growth seen during infancy. Most girls experience their growth spurt between ages 10 and 14, with an average annual height increase of 6–8 cm, typically less than boys. This rapid growth phase lasts approximately two years and includes a weight gain of about 2 kg annually.

Many girls experience bone and joint discomfort during this period, often called "growing pains." These pains, particularly common at night, can even precede the growth spurt. Warm baths, gentle massages, or soothing drinks like warm milk or tea often help alleviate the discomfort. Pain relievers are rarely necessary.

Is it possible to predict a girl's adult height? While the topic is debated, a commonly used formula among parents and doctors is:

Predicted height for girls = (Father's height + Mother's height) / 2 - 5 cm

Extremely rapid growth (over 10 cm per year) in girls older than 6–7 years, particularly if accompanied by other signs of early puberty, should prompt a medical evaluation to rule out underlying conditions.

Did You Know?

- *The average age of puberty onset in girls has decreased, with breast development now starting earlier due to factors like environmental pollution and diet.*
- *Girls typically experience a growth spurt between ages 10 and 14, growing 6–8 cm annually. " Growing pains " are a common symptom during this phase.*

Menarche

For centuries, menarche, the first menstrual period, was viewed as a key milestone marking the onset of puberty and a girl's readiness for childbearing. In many cultures, this milestone historically led to early marriages, often as young as 14–15, a practice common until the early 20th century.

Menarche typically occurs about two years after the larval (breast budding). Over the past century, the average age of menarche has decreased from around 14.5 to 12.5, and in some countries, it is now closer to 11.5.

The timing of menarche often follows a hereditary pattern, closely resembling that of the girl's mother or maternal grandmother. Approximately 60% of the variation in menarcheal timing and menstrual cycle characteristics is genetically determined. While specific genes influencing menarche have not been identified, genes related to progesterone receptor function are known to play a significant role.

Body weight and fat percentage are critical factors influencing the onset of menarche. To begin menstruating, a girl must typically reach a minimum body weight of around 48 kg, with body fat accounting for 17–22% of total body weight. Body fat is vital for processing and storing sex hormones.

A regular menstrual cycle does not establish itself immediately but develops gradually. Its regulation involves visible processes, such as ovulation and menstruation, and invisible hormonal fluctuations that begin long before menarche. A dedicated chapter discusses more detailed information about menstrual cycle development in adolescents.

Pubertal Development Disorders

Pubertal development disorders in girls typically fall into two main categories: **precocious puberty (PP)** and **delayed puberty (DP)**. Historically, these conditions were managed by various specialists, including psychiatrists, rather than gynecologists. This fragmented approach led to inconsistent and sometimes arbitrary standards for defining normal child development.

Precocious puberty has traditionally been defined as the appearance of secondary sexual characteristics, such as breast development or pubic hair, before the age of 8. However, modern research suggests that these changes may occur as early as ages 6–7 in some girls. As a result, current guidelines now classify the onset of secondary sexual characteristics before age seven as precocious in Caucasian girls and before age 6 in African girls.

Delayed puberty is typically defined as the absence of secondary sexual characteristics by ages 13–14 or a failure to menstruate within five years after the onset of breast development. Several additional factors are critical in evaluating pubertal development, including growth rate, height, and weight, symptoms involving the central nervous system, and behavioral changes. Reported prevalence rates for pubertal development disorders vary significantly worldwide, with 5–25% of girls experiencing early puberty, particularly in certain African regions where rates are notably higher.

Assessing normal pubertal development requires consideration of various external and internal factors, such as obesity, low socioeconomic status, emotional stress, and the absence of a biological father. These factors can influence not only the timing and duration of puberty but also the overall health and behavior of adolescents.

The precise relationship between the rise of gonadotropins, androgen levels, and the onset of menarche is not fully understood. Research suggests that external factors, including socioeconomic status, family dynamics, and body weight, have a profound impact on the timing of menarche and the emergence of secondary sexual characteristics. For example, obese girls tend to experience menarche approximately five months earlier than their average-weight peers, even when gonadotropin levels are similar. Conversely, in families with higher income or lower family conflict, androgen increases, and the onset of menstruation tends to occur later.

While certain puberty stages involve predictable hormonal changes, establishing a direct link between these hormonal shifts and the emergence of secondary sexual characteristics remains challenging. Factors such as genetics, chromosomal variations, chronic health conditions, and intense physical activity also play significant roles in determining puberty's pattern, timing, and duration.

The **Life History Theory** posits that infancy and early childhood experiences, along with their physical and psychological impacts, can shape pubertal development and influence a woman's long-term reproductive health.

Classification of Pubertal Development Disorders

Pubertal development disorders in girls are generally classified into the following categories:

Isosexual: Pubertal changes that align with the child's biological sex.
Heterosexual: The development of masculine traits or characteristics in girls.
True Precocious Puberty: Early activation of the hypothalamic-pituitary-gonadal axis, leading to the typical sequence of pubertal events occurring prematurely.

Pseudo-Precocious Puberty: The early appearance of secondary sexual characteristics due to factors other than the activation of the hypothalamic-pituitary-gonadal axis, such as hormone-secreting tumors or exogenous hormone exposure.

For parents, especially those without a medical background, identifying puberty-related disorders can be challenging. Even parents with general medical knowledge may find it difficult to assess these complex conditions without specialized guidance. Consulting a qualified specialist is essential for accurate diagnosis and appropriate management if any abnormalities in pubertal development are suspected.

Precocious Puberty (PP)

Precocious puberty (PP) is more extensively researched than delayed puberty, mainly because the early onset of secondary sexual characteristics often raises immediate concerns among parents. PP is classified into two main categories: **gonadotropin-dependent PP** (true or central PP) and **gonadotropin-independent PP**.

1. **Gonadotropin-Dependent PP**

Also referred to as true or central PP, this form is caused by the premature activation of the hypothalamic-pituitary-gonadal axis. This early activation triggers the release of hormones that typically initiate puberty, leading to hormonal imbalances originating in the pituitary gland.

1. **Gonadotropin-Independent PP**

This type is known as peripheral or pseudo-precocious puberty, which results from conditions unrelated to the hypothalamic-pituitary axis. It is often linked to disorders affecting the adrenal glands, such as **congenital adrenal hyperplasia** or tumors that produce gonadotropins (e.g., human chorionic gonadotropin, or hCG). Other potential causes include adrenal tumors, ovarian tumors, and specific syndromes.

Some cases of PP are genetically influenced, often inherited in an autosomal dominant pattern. This form, known as constitutional or familial PP, is typically idiopathic (of unknown cause) and is the most common subtype of gonadotropin-independent PP.

Notably, in 8–33% of cases, precocious puberty is associated with brain and central nervous system abnormalities, including tumors and congenital malformations. This highlights the importance of a thorough medical evaluation to rule out severe underlying conditions when early puberty is suspected.

PP can manifest in two distinct forms: complete and partial.

- Complete PP: This form follows the typical sequence of secondary sexual characteristic development, mirroring normal puberty but occurring at an unusually early age.
- Partial PP: This form involves isolated or incomplete signs of puberty, such as:
    - **Premature Thelarche**: Early development of breast tissue without other signs of puberty.
    - **Premature Adrenarche**: Early growth of pubic or underarm hair, often due to elevated androgen levels.
    - **Premature Menarche**: The early onset of menstruation without the expected sequence of other pubertal changes.

These classifications guide healthcare providers in identifying the underlying causes of precocious puberty and determining the most appropriate course of treatment. Early diagnosis and intervention are crucial to addressing potential complications and ensuring the child's well-being.

Signs of Precocious Puberty in Girls: Key Indicators

Precocious puberty (PP) presents several signs requiring monitoring and evaluation. Common indicators include:

- Accelerated growth and early weight gain
- Bone age advanced by more than two years

- Breast development before ages 7–8
- Appearance of pubic or underarm hair before ages 7–8
- Vaginal bleeding or early menstruation
- Uterine enlargement
- Neurological symptoms such as headaches, fatigue, or vision problems

If these signs are observed, a pediatric gynecologist should evaluate the child. The assessment should include a detailed medical history, including the mother's pregnancy, the family's medical background, and the child's growth and development records.

Diagnosing PP often involves laboratory tests to measure hormone levels, including luteinizing hormone (LH), follicle-stimulating hormone (FSH), human chorionic gonadotropin (hCG), estradiol, thyroid hormones (TSH and T4), insulin, and glucose. Imaging studies such as X-rays (for skeletal bone age), MRI (to evaluate the brain and pituitary gland), ultrasound (of the ovaries and uterus), and karyotyping (to check for chromosomal abnormalities) can provide additional insights.

The treatment of PP depends on the underlying cause and includes:

- Medical Management: Hormonal therapy to delay further progression and manage symptoms.
- Surgical Intervention: Required in cases involving ovarian, adrenal, or brain tumors.
- Psychotherapy: Support for emotional and psychological challenges associated with early puberty.

In cases of mild or isolated increases in breast tissue or early pubic hair development before ages 7–8, observation may suffice. Extensive testing or intervention is often unnecessary unless symptoms progress.

Partial Precocious Puberty

Partial PP involves isolated signs of puberty without full development. Common forms include:

1. **Precocious Thelarche**

Early breast development before age 3. Hormonal levels are typically normal, and breast tissue often regresses without intervention within 2–4 years. Monitoring is usually sufficient.

2. **Precocious Adrenarche**

The early appearance of pubic or underarm hair is associated with elevated levels of weak androgens (DHEA, DHEAS). This condition is generally identified through lab tests before ages 5–6 and may include slightly advanced bone age. Treatment is rarely required.

3. **Precocious Menarche**

Isolated vaginal bleeding without other secondary sexual characteristics. This may be due to trauma, inflammation, foreign objects, or medical conditions like thyroid dysfunction or ovarian tumors. Diagnosing the cause and ruling out other issues, such as sexual trauma, is critical. Vaginal bleeding typically resolves within 1–2 years without treatment.

Delayed Puberty in Girls: Key Points

Delayed puberty often goes unnoticed by parents, as teens may hide symptoms or be unaware of developmental delays. Signs of delayed puberty include:

- No breast development by ages 13–14
- Absence of menstruation by age 16 or within five years after the onset of breast development
- Lack of pubic hair by ages 14–15

Delayed puberty can result from several causes and is classified as follows:

1. **Genetic and Chromosomal Factors**

Conditions such as Turner syndrome, Noonan syndrome, or constitutional delay.

2. **Chronic Illnesses**

Chronic diseases like diabetes, inflammatory bowel disease, cystic fibrosis, or kidney disease can delay puberty.

3. **Induced Causes**

Factors like chemotherapy, radiation therapy, or intense athletic training can suppress hormonal development.

Family-related delays and malnutrition (e.g., anorexia, bulimia, or chronic neglect) are significant contributors to delayed puberty. Studies suggest that early childhood neglect, abuse, or poor care from birth to age seven can influence the timing of puberty.

Most cases of delayed puberty resolve with lifestyle adjustments, such as improving nutrition, reducing strenuous physical activity, and ensuring adequate rest. Psychotherapy may help address emotional challenges, while supportive hormonal therapy might be necessary in some cases.

Each case of delayed puberty is unique and requires an individualized treatment plan. Parents and healthcare providers should avoid a one-size-fits-all approach and focus instead on the child's specific needs for optimal outcomes.

Recommendations for Parents Regarding Pubertal Development Disorders

1. **Educate Yourself About Normal Pubertal Timelines**

   Understand the typical age ranges for pubertal milestones, such as breast development, growth spurts, and menarche, to differentiate between normal variations and potential disorders.

2. **Monitor Growth and Development**

   Keep track of your child's height, weight, and physical changes. Look for early signs of puberty, such as breast budding or pubic hair growth before age 8, or delayed signs, such as no breast development by age 13-14.

3. **Address Nutritional and Lifestyle Factors**

   Provide a balanced diet rich in essential nutrients and ensure regular physical activity. Avoid diets that lead to extreme weight gain or loss, as obesity and malnutrition can impact pubertal timing.

4. **Encourage Open Communication**

Create a safe and supportive environment where your child feels comfortable discussing physical and emotional changes.

5. **Be Vigilant for Emotional or Behavioral Changes**

   Look for signs of emotional stress or behavioral shifts that might indicate underlying issues related to early or delayed puberty.

6. **Seek Professional Guidance**

   If you notice signs of precocious or delayed puberty, consult a specialist, such as a pediatric endocrinologist or gynecologist, for evaluation and management.

Did You Know?

- *A girl's development often mirrors her mother's or maternal grandmother's patterns, with genetics accounting for about 60% of pubertal timing.*
- *Chronic illnesses, hormonal imbalances, or malnutrition may go unnoticed until delayed puberty raises concerns, highlighting the importance of regular monitoring.*

The Menstrual Cycle

One of the most pervasive misunderstandings in gynecology, held by many women and even some healthcare providers, is the belief that menstruation itself is the primary indicator of a normal menstrual cycle. This misconception leads to countless misdiagnoses and inappropriate treatments. Much like philosophical debates about the primacy of matter versus consciousness, menstruation is not the central determinant of reproductive potential in reproductive health.

The true foundation of the menstrual cycle lies in the maturation of ovarian egg cells (oocytes).

Menstruation, on the other hand, is merely a secondary, confirmatory sign that pregnancy has not occurred.

Another common misunderstanding surrounds the definition of a "regular" menstrual cycle. Many women mistakenly assume that any deviation from the "ideal" 28-day cycle described in textbooks or popular literature signals a problem. This belief often drives them to seek medical advice for minor delays, early menstruation, or cycles that do not align perfectly with this perceived standard. Mothers may even bring their teenage daughters to the doctor because their early menstrual cycles lack consistency, not realizing that irregularity is a natural part of adolescence.

Equally misunderstood is the idea that irregular menstrual cycles are consistently abnormal. There are natural periods throughout life when cycles are expected to be irregular. Adolescence, for instance, is a time when hormonal systems are still maturing, making irregular cycles familiar. Numerous factors, many overlooked or misunderstood by women and some doctors, can influence menstrual cycles.

These misconceptions about the female body are often passed down through generations, from mothers to daughters, older sisters to younger ones, and aunts to nieces. It perpetuates a cycle of misinformation that affects how women view and manage their reproductive health.

What happens when a teenage girl doesn't experience the mythical "perfect" 28-day cycle? Frequently, she is taken to a doctor and prescribed hormonal contraceptives, often older-generation formulations. They are given at a time when her menstrual regulatory system is still developing and usually continues for months or even years. It creates a harmful cycle: while taking hormones, her periods appear regular, but once she stops, irregularity resumes, leading to repeated prescriptions for hormonal treatment.

Understanding the menstrual cycle and addressing these misconceptions is vital for women and the next generation. Sharing accurate, evidence-based information can empower girls to understand their bodies better, avoid unnecessary interventions, and foster a healthier relationship with their reproductive health.

This knowledge is essential and should be shared with your daughters.

What is the role of a woman from Nature's perspective?

To understand the role menstrual cycles play in a woman's life, we should start with a fundamental question: What is a woman's role from Nature's viewpoint?

In biology, humans are classified as the highest representatives of the animal kingdom, belonging to the class of mammals and the primate order. While some may feel uncomfortable equating humans with animals, let alone "primates," the reality is that our bodies are governed by the same natural laws that apply to all living organisms. These laws, whether attributed to Nature, God, or another belief system, dictate how our bodies are structured and function.

Life depends on reproduction, and humans are no exception. Offspring represent the continuation of life, ensuring the survival of a unique species. Like all animals, humans progress through distinct phases: birth, growth and maturation, reproductive maturity, and eventual aging.

Humans, however, have the unique ability to choose whether to reproduce. Despite this choice, Nature's processes remain constant, and life unfolds according to its inherent laws. When we examine a girl's journey from birth through puberty, it becomes clear that this is a natural progression, a self-replication program embedded in our genes and brain functions.

Reproduction requires specific components: reproductive cells, conditions for conception, and the capacity to nurture developing offspring. Carrying and bearing children is a role Nature has uniquely assigned to women. To fulfill this role, women have ovaries to store and mature reproductive cells (oocytes), fallopian tubes where fertilization occurs, a uterus to nourish and support the developing child, and a vagina to receive male reproductive cells and serve as the birth canal during childbirth.

The reproductive period, commonly called the **reproductive age**, typically spans about 15 to 50 years. During this time, women usually experience menstrual cycles, but it is essential to understand that menstruation alone does not determine a woman's ability to conceive. Ovulation, the process in which a mature oocyte is released, is the critical factor. Without ovulation, conception is not possible, even if menstruation occurs. Conversely, conception can still happen in the absence of menstruation under certain conditions.

The number of yearly ovulations a healthy woman experiences varies, primarily depending on her age and other contributing factors. When puberty begins, it triggers the onset of reproductive function, initially marked by irregular hormonal surges and attempts at follicular maturation in the ovaries. Over time, these irregular patterns stabilize, eventually leading to the regular, well-defined menstrual cycles that characterize reproductive maturity.

Understanding these processes reveals how intricately the menstrual cycle and reproductive function are designed as part of Nature's overarching plan for life.

What is the Menstrual Cycle?

If we define the primary distinction between women of reproductive age and other age groups, it would be the presence of menstruation — visible as blood-tinged vaginal discharge. This discharge is something a woman can observe, making its absence an indicator of pregnancy or other factors disrupting the cycle.

In medicine, however, the menstrual cycle is more accurately defined not by the bleeding days but by the egg maturation process. When analyzing reproductive health or employing reproductive technologies, the cycle is often measured from ovulation or, more precisely, from the pre-ovulatory surge in luteinizing hormone (LH) in the blood. This surge is imperceptible without laboratory testing, and ovulation cannot be confirmed without additional examination. For practical reasons, menstruation has become the known marker of the cycle's start.

The menstrual cycle is the body's monthly preparation for accepting a fertilized egg. In the first half of the cycle, egg cells mature. In the second half, if conception occurs, the fertilized egg implants in the uterus, and pregnancy begins. If conception does not occur, the last week of the cycle focuses on shedding the unused, built-up endometrium, resulting in menstruation.

Although referring to menstruation as "critical days" has become popular recently, this terminology is misleading. Historically, "critical days" referred to the period in the middle of the cycle when ovulation typically occurs, days when conception is most likely. Identifying the exact moment of ovulation is complex, but women can learn to recognize signs of its approach. These days were once termed "critical" due to their significance in achieving or avoiding pregnancy.

Teaching these physiological processes to a girl, especially a teenager, can be challenging, but it is fundamental to understanding reproductive health. This knowledge is essential for maintaining well-being and preventing misconceptions that could lead to serious mistakes for mothers and their daughters, the future women who may one day wish to become mothers themselves.

Why 28 Days?

In ancient times, people lacked knowledge about ovarian structures or the mechanisms regulating ovulation and the menstrual cycle, but they recognized the cyclical Nature of female reproduction. The menstrual cycle was revered, celebrated in rituals, and deeply connected to cultural and spiritual beliefs.

Many cultures worshipped the moon, as its phases were thought to mirror the menstrual cycle. The word "menstruation" itself is derived from the Latin word for "moon" and the Greek word for "month." The average cycle length of 28 days is coincidentally close to the lunar month, though there is no direct relationship between the phases of the moon and the menstrual cycle. Nonetheless, myths and associations between the two persist.

Even today, pregnancy is measured in obstetric months, each equal to 28 days or one lunar cycle. A full-term pregnancy lasts about 280 days or 10 lunar months. Before the Julian calendar, the pregnancy term was calculated using lunar months, and this tradition continues in some cultural practices. Modern obstetrics prefers counting pregnancy in weeks to avoid confusion between lunar and calendar months.

28 is symbolic in many cultures, often regarded as ideal or fortunate. Many ancient calendars, except the Egyptian one, were lunar rather than solar. This cultural attachment to the number 28 is like the fixation on 36.6°C as the ideal body temperature, another generalized standard that doesn't reflect the variability of real-life biology.

In reality, menstrual cycles fluctuate and are rarely a perfect 28 days. There are no women whose cycles have never deviated from the textbook "ideal." Early or delayed cycles are common and entirely natural.

Menstrual Cycle: Essential Facts to Know

Much has been written about menstruation and the menstrual cycle, including me in my books (*Hormone Therapy in Obstetrics and Gynecology: Myths and Realities; Hormonal Intelligence: How Hormones Shape Health and Well-being; When you are ready; Baby, are you coming?; 1000 + questions and answers on gynecology*). To avoid repetition, here are the essential facts about the menstrual cycle in summarized form:

- The menstrual cycle is classically divided into two phases. The first phase, known as the **estrogenic**, **proliferative**, or **pre-ovulatory phase**, involves the maturation of the follicle (egg cell). The second phase, the **progesterone**, **secretory**, or **luteal phase**, prepares the uterus to accept a fertilized egg and support the onset of pregnancy.
- These phases do not establish immediately after menarche; they require several years to mature. In adolescents, especially during the first years of menstrual cycles, many cycles are anovulatory (do not involve egg maturation).
- A menstrual cycle lasting between **21 and 35 days**, with up to a **7-day variation in either direction**, is considered normal. However, cycles may be longer and irregular in adolescents up to ages 21–22.
- Menstruation can be described as the **shedding of the uterus**, resulting from the detachment of the old uterine lining (endometrium) and its replacement with a new one.
- The endometrium is a dynamic tissue that undergoes constant changes based on the menstrual cycle phase.
- The endometrium consists of two layers:

- The **functional layer** detaches during menstruation.
- The **basal layer** is from which the new functional layer regenerates. Damage to the basal layer can cause menstrual disturbances and infertility.

❖ Before menstruation begins, hormone levels in the body drop to very low levels, triggering the detachment of the endometrium. This results in menstruation, also known as **physiological withdrawal bleeding from hormones**.

❖ The shedding of the endometrium is not instantaneous; it begins in specific areas and continues over **4-5 days**. During this time, regeneration of the endometrium also starts.

❖ Menstrual blood does not contain clots. What women often perceive as clots are **small fragments of the detached endometrium**.

Did You Know?

- *Menstrual cycles don't always follow the "perfect" 28-day rule—cycles between 21 and 35 days are considered normal, especially in adolescents.*
- *Menstruation is not the primary indicator of reproductive health; ovulation is central to determining fertility.*

Do Adolescents Have Ovulation?

When an adult woman visits a doctor with concerns about irregular menstrual cycles or difficulty conceiving, the first step is to determine whether ovulation is occurring. **Ovulation, the maturation of egg cells, is fundamental to a healthy menstrual cycle and reproductive function**. However, a common misconception among many doctors is that once a teenage girl begins menstruating, all her cycles must be ovulatory.

Even in healthy adult women, not every cycle is ovulatory. Younger women (under 21–22) and older women (over 30-32) are more likely to experience anovulatory (non-ovulatory) cycles. Additionally, various factors can influence the menstrual cycle, a topic discussed in detail in this book.

When does ovulation begin in adolescents? Does the first menstruation involve ovulation, and how frequently do adolescents ovulate? What happens with hormone levels before menarche and during the early years of menstrual development?

Research has shown that adolescent girls may experience frequent progesterone surges before menarche. This phenomenon was initially challenging to understand due to the difficulty of adequately monitoring adolescents (this monitoring requires frequent blood sampling to measure hormone levels).

Studies indicate that about 12% of adolescent girls (average age 12) exhibit hormonal fluctuations typical of an ovulatory pattern, suggesting that ovulation could occur before the first menstruation. However, these findings were not confirmed through ultrasound examination. All adolescent girls show elevated levels of testosterone, estradiol, and 17-hydroxyprogesterone, with girls displaying ovulatory hormone surges having even higher levels.

Further research reveals that **the first menstruation is not accompanied by ovulation** in most adolescents. However, the rise in luteinizing hormone (LH) and progesterone levels before menarche in some girls explains rare cases of pregnancy occurring in adolescents before the onset of menstruation.

Menarche does not depend on ethnicity or race but is influenced by the child's weight (body mass index). Establishing regular ovulatory cycles takes several years—on average, 5–7 years. Thus, until ages 20–22, many young women may experience cycles without egg maturation multiple times a year.

Another common misconception among women and even some doctors is that ovaries function alternately, with ovulation occurring in one ovary one month and in the other the next. If ovulation is observed via ultrasound in the same ovary over three cycles, it is often mistakenly assumed that only one ovary functions. In reality, the sequence of ovulation between the ovaries is **unpredictable**. Ovulation may occur several times in a row in the same ovary, which is normal. However, ovulation is more commonly observed in the right ovary. This does not mean the other ovary is "not functioning." Exceptions occur when a significant portion of one ovary is removed (e.g., during surgery for a tumor), leaving only its stroma (supportive tissue) with minimal or no follicular apparatus.

Attempts to "force" such damaged ovaries to function through stimulation methods can cause harm.

For teenage girls with irregular menstrual cycles, inconsistent ovulation is regular and does not require treatment, especially with hormones. Understanding this natural developmental phase helps avoid unnecessary medical interventions.

Establishment of the Menstrual Cycle in Adolescence

Over the past 150 years, the age at which girls begin menstruating has significantly decreased. The average age of menarche (the first menstrual period) depends on factors such as race, nutrition, urban or rural living conditions, heredity, body weight, and other influences. Thirty years ago, the average age of menarche in many countries was approximately 14.5 years. Today, it has dropped to about 12.4 years. Around 10% of girls begin menstruating by age 11, 90% by age 13.8, and 98% by age 15.

As the menstrual cycle begins to establish itself during adolescence, its characteristics differ from those of adult women. Numerous studies have documented menstrual cycle patterns and irregularities in adolescents over the past three decades. For 38% of girls, the interval between menarche and the second menstruation exceeds 40 days; for 10%, it is over 60 days; and for 20%, it is only 20 days. The first menstruation typically ranges from 2 to 7 days but can sometimes extend up to 2 weeks.

In the first three years following menarche, menstrual cycles are often longer than the typical 28-35 days seen in adults. Over time, cycles become shorter, more regular, and more frequently accompanied by ovulation. The following patterns are considered normal for adolescents:

- First-year after menarche: 23-90 days (average 32 days);
- Fourth year: 24-50 days;
- Seventh year: 27-38 days.

Regular cycles generally do not establish themselves until approximately 18 months after the first menstruation. After two years, cycles often become regular and ovulatory; however, 50% of adolescents experience anovulation during the first three years after menarche. The later menarche occurs, the longer it takes for ovulatory cycles to establish.

In anovulatory cycles, ovulation does not occur, meaning the cycle phases are absent.

Diagnosing progesterone deficiency or luteal insufficiency (luteal phase deficiency) in such cases is incorrect, and treatment with progesterone medications is entirely unwarranted.

Adolescents often experience a shortened luteal phase in ovulatory cycles, but cycle duration can vary significantly compared to adults. It is important for parents, especially mothers, to understand that despite variability in cycle length and irregularity, ovulatory cycles may still occur (though not always).

An individual's menstrual cycle typically stabilizes fully around ages 19-20. Menstruation lasts 3-7 days, and girls generally use 3-6 pads per day.

Parents and adolescent girls need to understand that the establishment of menstrual cycles is a highly individual process, differing for each girl. Hormone levels, cycle length, and ovulation patterns should not be compared to adult women.

Even in adults, menstrual cycle regularity is influenced by numerous factors, which will be explored further in this book.

Factors Affecting the Menstrual Cycle

According to the philosophical principle of cause and effect, every phenomenon (effect) must have a reason. This cause is not always immediately apparent or explainable, not because it does not exist, but because various obstacles and limitations hinder complete understanding.

The human body is an extraordinarily complex creation of Nature, consisting of billions of cells, millions of chemical reactions, and thousands of chemical substances, all intricately interconnected. These components function autonomously and in relation to other structures within the body. Beyond the physical, humans possess consciousness and thought, which can influence bodily functions and potentially lead to deviations that manifest as diseases. The familiar adage "all diseases come from nerves" reflects a profound truth, especially about the reproductive system.

In addition to direct causes of disease, there are factors that "activate" these causes. These can be numerous and varied. Some, known as risk factors, have been linked to certain diseases through medical research. Others act as incidental triggers, sometimes in combination, creating conditions for problems to arise.

The formation and regularity of the menstrual cycle are influenced by a wide range of internal (within the body) and external (environmental) factors. However, the most significant determinant is the individual's response to events - how a woman or girl perceives her body, surroundings, interpersonal relationships, and life experiences. The more negative the reaction, particularly if it is accompanied by fear or other intense emotions, the greater the likelihood of health issues.

Emerging research has revealed the significant impact of environmental pollutants on the timing of puberty. Endocrine-disrupting chemicals (EDCs), such as bisphenol A (BPA) and phthalates, mimic or block natural hormones, leading to hormonal imbalances. Exposure to EDCs during critical developmental windows has been associated with early puberty in girls, characterized by premature thelarche or menarche. Conversely, some pollutants, like persistent organic pollutants (POPs), may delay puberty by interfering with the hypothalamic-pituitary-gonadal axis. Understanding these effects highlights the need for stricter regulations on EDC exposure and increased awareness among parents about minimizing environmental risks.

Humans can be compared to highly advanced computers, running genetic "programs" coded in their DNA. The brain acts as the central control system, overseeing the execution of these programs while continuously analyzing and interpreting signals from both the body and the external environment. Even thoughts act as signals, capable of influencing bodily functions, particularly the more primitive brain regions where centers of self-preservation and regulation are located.

Is There a Program of Self-Destruction? It appears so. One of the most alarming and enigmatic conditions that can emerge in an otherwise healthy body due to a profound psychological conflict with body image is anorexia. This condition, discussed further in other chapters, exemplifies the destructive power of the mind over physical health. Anorexia is notoriously difficult to treat, and its most devastating outcome occurs when a self-destructive mechanism within the body is activated. At this stage, no dietary interventions, medical treatments, or even positive psychological shifts seem capable of reversing the damage. The mortality rate associated with anorexia remains tragically high.

This highlights the importance of raising children without instilling excessive fear or exaggerating situations that can be managed without professional intervention. Teaching children how to process and respond to adverse events, whether in their own lives or the lives of others, is essential for fostering resilience and emotional balance.

With this understanding of the body's interconnected systems, it becomes clear that, in many cases, women inadvertently contribute to menstrual cycle disturbances due to a lack of knowledge about what is expected and what constitutes a deviation. Unfortunately, these vital lessons are seldom part of formal education at any level, and few individuals proactively seek answers to questions like, "How is my body structured, and how does it function?"

When noticeable deviations occur, fear often overwhelms rational thought, hindering the ability to assess the situation calmly. By addressing the underlying factors that influence the menstrual cycle, we can empower women with the knowledge to understand their bodies better and take informed actions

- **Age**

It is a well-established fact that menstrual cycles in teenage girls are irregular, and that speaks volumes. Expecting perfectly regular cycles before the ages of 21-22 is unrealistic, given the fluctuations in body weight, rapid growth, and heightened sensitivity to stress. Adolescents and young women often struggle to process life events without intense emotional responses, including fear, worry, or tears. With limited experience in resilience and tolerance, their idealism usually leads to extreme reactions, affecting not just their mental state but also their physical development. It's critical to avoid comparing the processes occurring in a teenager's body to those of an adult woman.

The most common combination impacting menstrual cycle regularity in teenagers can be described as the "teenage triad": *young age, low or high weight, and a pronounced adverse reaction to stress.*

- **Energy Balance and Metabolism**

While it's simpler to discuss "weight issues," it's far more critical to explain to women, particularly adolescents, that menstrual irregularities often stem from an energy imbalance. The body's healthy functioning relies on the exchange of energy derived from nutrient metabolism. However, energy balance is not determined solely by the quantity and quality of food consumed.

For instance, consuming a bottle of vodka or whiskey does not provide the necessary kilocalories, despite this alarming trend among teens who turn to alcohol out of a misguided fear of gaining weight. This has fueled a growing problem of teenage alcoholism worldwide.

In addition to nutrition, physical activity, and emotional well-being significantly influence energy metabolism.

During adolescence, synthetic processes dominate as the body grows rapidly. Weight gain and heightened metabolism are natural during this stage, as energy use is at its peak. As a girl nears the end of puberty, her metabolism slows and stabilizes between 20 and 26. After this period, metabolic processes gradually decelerate, with the onset of aging accelerating closer to age 40, often beginning subtly around 35-37 years old.

Energy imbalances are rare with a healthy lifestyle, as the mature body is capable of compensating for minor disruptions. Even in cases of significant energy loss, the body's compensatory mechanisms, provided there are no underlying illnesses, effectively restore balance.

Teenagers, however, are especially vulnerable to societal pressures, often developing "inferiority complexes" influenced by media portrayals of idealized beauty. Celebrities and influencers in entertainment, cinema, and sports promote unrealistic body standards that deeply affect young girls' self-perception. The image of the "ideal woman" has shifted dramatically over the last century and even within the last few decades. For example, the Mona Lisa would likely be mocked today for her pale complexion, lack of makeup, and rounded features. At the same time, the full-bodied figures celebrated in Rubens' and Raphael's works would never qualify for modern modeling standards.

Both acute and chronic illnesses can significantly disrupt energy balance. These imbalances are most pronounced in cases involving endocrine disorders that impair hormone production, metabolic diseases that affect nutrient absorption, exhausting chronic conditions of any kind, and physical depletion.

The brain is the first organ to respond to an energy shortage, as it requires a steady supply of glucose—its primary energy source. Additionally, optimal blood flow and oxygen levels are crucial for brain function, which is maintained through physical and mental activity.

In situations of energy imbalance, the body activates self-preservation mechanisms, redistributing energy and oxygen to prioritize vital organs. The brain and heart receive top priority, while secondary organs like the kidneys, liver, and gastrointestinal tract see reduced resource allocation. Being the least critical for immediate survival, the reproductive system is the first to experience functional decline, with processes like egg maturation slowing or halting entirely.

In women, reproduction depends on the maturation of egg cells, reflected in menstrual cycles. In an energy crisis, the body naturally eliminates the additional burden of pregnancy, as carrying a fetus — essentially a "foreign organism" — demands significant energy and nutrients. Consequently, the maturation of egg cells slows or stops, and menstrual cycles either cease or become infrequent and prolonged. If ovulation ceases entirely, menstruation stops, acting as an additional self-preservation mechanism to avoid minimal blood loss (usually no more than 50-80 ml per cycle).

This self-preservation strategy applies universally, from the onset of menstruation to menopause. However, puberty is the most vulnerable period, as the processes governing reproductive function are still developing. Unfortunately, these mechanisms can sometimes become irreversible. Since the exact methods for disabling and restoring reproductive function are not fully understood, interventions remain limited and challenging.

- **Body Structure**

The balance of body proportions, height, and weight is intricately linked to energy balance and metabolism. While women may differ in height and weight, the critical factor is the proportion or weight-to-height ratio. A shorter woman may appear heavier, while the same weight in a taller woman might be considered normal or even low.

Earlier, a child's weight was not a significant concern in predicting future health outcomes. However, with the dramatic rise in obesity among both children and adults, this has become a critical focus.

Much research has been conducted on obesity's impact on menstrual cycles, though most studies center on adult women. In such cases, obesity is often associated with irregular menstrual cycles, infertility, and pregnancy loss. Fat tissue is a reservoir for male sex hormones, which can indirectly affect egg maturation.

In adolescents, however, excess weight has less of a negative impact on the onset of menstruation and the establishment of regular cycles compared to weight deficiency. It is not solely about weight but rather the weight-to-height ratio.

A short girl may suffer from obesity, while the same weight in a taller girl may be considered normal or even low. To assess this proportion, many rely on a simple formula for calculating "ideal" weight: subtract 100 from the height in centimeters. For example, a girl with a height of 165 cm would have an ideal weight of 65 kg.

However, this method is not entirely accurate. Deviations of up to 10% in either direction are considered normal. For a height of 165 cm, this translates to a weight range of 58.5–71.5 kg. While this formula provides a quick reference, it applies more to adult women. Growth and weight charts are better tools for determining optimal weight for growing children and adolescents.

The Body Mass Index (BMI) is another commonly used measure, calculated as body weight (kg) divided by height (m^2). A BMI between 20 and 24.9 is considered normal, 25–29.9 indicates overweight (Grade I obesity), 30–40 indicates Grade II obesity, and over 40 indicates Grade III obesity. A BMI below 20 is also considered abnormal. While BMI is traditionally used for adults, there are now age-specific BMI tables for children and adolescents.

In recent years, discussions about women's health have increasingly highlighted the role of body fat percentage. Various methods and formulas exist for calculating body fat, with different parameters used in fields such as sports and medicine. Often, the body fat levels considered optimal for athletes are not aligned with what is deemed healthy from a medical perspective.

Studies have shown that the onset of menarche (the first menstrual period) requires at least 17% body fat relative to a teenager's total weight. For menstrual cycles to become regular, body fat should reach around 21–24%. Girls with a low weight-to-height ratio typically experience delayed menarche and require more time for their cycles to stabilize.

In contrast, adolescents with obesity tend to develop menstrual irregularities later, after the completion of puberty. This underscores the importance of maintaining a healthy balance in body proportions, as underweight and overweight conditions can influence the development and regularity of menstrual cycles.

- **Stress and Emotionality**

Fifteen to twenty years ago, the term "stress" was seldom discussed in scientific or medical literature and was rarely mentioned in popular media. Today, even children are familiar with the word. But what do doctors mean by stress? Can the age-old saying, "all diseases come from nerves," be rephrased as "all diseases come from stress"? The answer is yes. Stress responses are reactions to external and internal stimuli intricately linked to the nervous system, including the brain.

Stress can be defined in many ways, but at its core, it is a reaction to a stressor – any stimulus or event. This reaction is intensely individual, depending on how a person perceives a disruption to their equilibrium, whether energetic or emotional. Such a shift can result in either positive or adverse effects.

Interestingly, people tend to focus less on positive stress and more on negative stress. Negative stress is often tied to emotions such as fear, confusion, insecurity, aggression, anger, and disappointment. For some individuals, a stressful situation can be a positive motivator, driving action and improvement. For others, it is an opposing force, causing inaction, apathy, panic, or hysteria.

Children learn to respond to events through their parents' behaviors and reactions, often adopting similar responses. For example, if a mother panics whenever her child steps into a puddle, the child may associate puddles or cold water with fear. Over time, this could lead to avoidance behaviors, such as refusing to walk barefoot or worrying about cold feet causing illness.

A girl's reaction to significant and often private events in her life, such as puberty and menstruation, is frequently influenced by her mother's experiences, which may not always have been positive. When mothers project their past struggles or fears onto their daughters, it can lead to misunderstandings and unnecessary distress for both.

Short-term acute stress typically has minimal long-term impact on a child's health, especially if they have supportive parents. However, tragic events—such as the loss of a parent, friend, or other loved one—can profoundly affect a child's behavior and physiological processes. In such cases, seeking professional help from a psychologist, psychotherapist, or pediatrician is highly recommended.

Chronic stress, on the other hand, presents a more serious challenge. When adverse events persist for weeks, months, or even years, they can significantly affect health, particularly for a growing girl. Stress can originate from various sources, including physical (e.g., intensive sports), energetic (related to energy imbalance), psycho-emotional, or moral challenges. Regardless of the cause, prolonged stress can leave lasting effects on the body.

Research consistently highlights stress as a primary cause of irregular egg maturation (anovulation) and menstrual cycle disturbances, accounting for up to 70% of cases in adult women. This type of anovulation, often referred to as hypothalamic anovulation, points to the role of the hypothalamus in regulating human responses and behaviors, particularly those influenced by fear, aggression, and negative emotions. Stress-induced disruptions in hypothalamic activity can lead to imbalances in the production of substances that stimulate gonadotropin production by the pituitary gland.

For adolescent girls, whose emotional responses to challenges are often heightened and whose hypothalamic-pituitary system is still maturing, stress-related menstrual disturbances can be even more pronounced than in adult women. Recognizing the impact of stress and addressing it early is essential for fostering healthy physical and emotional development during adolescence.

- **Cognitive Function**

Cognition encompasses receiving, transforming, analyzing, and storing information from the environment and one's body. In simpler terms, it is how a person reacts to and interprets events. Every individual is unique, yet their behavior often follows predictable patterns. It's easy to understand that positive events generally evoke positive emotions. However, under intense or prolonged stress, reactions can become unpredictable, leading to fear, aggression, or even a loss of self-control.

A child's cognitive development is significantly influenced by the people they interact with most frequently, those they view as authority figures or even those they fear. Adolescence is a highly "emotional" phase of life, characterized by rapid mood swings and heightened sensitivity. Factors that seem insignificant to an adult can feel monumental to a teenager.

When a girl begins to experience the first signs of puberty, she often accepts these changes without much notice. However, as menstruation starts, along with early crushes and peer discussions about "taboo topics," she may begin to pay closer attention to her body. At this stage, concerns about uneven breast sizes, hair growth in unwanted areas, differences in the size of the labia minora, "extra" weight, or stretch marks on the thighs or chest may arise.

If a girl is unprepared for these "imperfections" and doesn't understand that they are normal and common, her reaction may be adverse, often fueled by a fear of being "abnormal." Such concerns can contribute to stress, potentially disrupting her menstrual cycle. Moreover, attempts at extreme dieting to address perceived body issues can lead to energy imbalances, further exacerbating reproductive health problems.

Open communication with children is essential. Explaining the origins of bodily changes, supporting them through challenging moments, and encouraging their initiative and creativity can significantly shape their self-perception and emotional resilience.

Having "heart-to-heart" conversations with their mothers can be particularly impactful for girls. These discussions foster a healthy response to menstrual cycle development and influence their future attitudes toward family and reproductive health.

Even when menstrual cycles are irregular, a mother's understanding and clear explanations of possible causes can make a significant difference. Such support enhances the likelihood of successful treatment, helps prevent recurring disruptions, and builds the girl's confidence and understanding of her body.

- **Daily and Annual Rhythms**

The influence of daily and annual rhythms, circadian and circannual rhythms, on the menstrual cycle is rarely discussed in detail, even in popular literature. However, many are familiar with biological rhythms or daily cycles.

Human bodies operate on alternating periods of wakefulness and rest, commonly known as activity and sleep cycles. These rhythms are present even in a fetus. By 28 weeks of pregnancy, a fetus develops distinct movement and sleep patterns. Toward the end of pregnancy, these alternate between light (surface-level) and deep sleep phases, lasting 70–90 minutes, independent of the mother's activity or time of day.

After birth, infants adjust to a day-night cycle over the first weeks and months of life, gradually forming their circadian rhythm. Before puberty, there is little connection between these rhythms and the substances regulating reproductive function. However, as a girl grows, the relationship between daily rhythms and menstrual cycles strengthens, sometimes referred to as daily changes across the menstrual cycle.

Daily rhythms manifest in fluctuations in body temperature, hormone production, and behavior, including activity and sleep patterns. Studies suggest that circadian rhythms also influence egg maturation (ovulation). For example, women working irregular shifts, such as night shifts, are more likely to experience menstrual irregularities and mood disturbances.

Hormones like melatonin and cortisol show significant circadian variation, especially during the second phase of the menstrual cycle. Melatonin, critical for sleep regulation, often declines in this phase, with many girls and women reporting sleep disturbances near the end of their cycle. Cortisol, the stress hormone, increases during this time, contributing to irritability, mood swings, and tearfulness. These changes often exacerbate insomnia and other sleep disruptions, highlighting the intricate relationship between circadian rhythms and the menstrual cycle.

The interaction is bidirectional: circadian rhythms can affect the monthly cycle, and menstrual cycles can influence circadian patterns.

On the other hand, annual rhythms are more prominent in animals, manifesting through migration, mating seasons, and varying activity levels (such as hibernation). Humans are not immune to these seasonal effects. Ovarian activity peaks during the summer, while anovulatory cycles are more frequent in winter. Spring often brings reports of menstrual irregularities, and premenstrual symptoms, including mood changes and depression, are more common in autumn and winter.

While some attribute these seasonal changes to reduced physical activity or less time spent outdoors in winter, the reality is more complex. Physical activity levels minimally influence these symptoms and are likely tied to broader biological rhythms.

In girls and young women, menstrual cycle patterns are influenced by a unique combination of factors, including daily and annual rhythms. These influences often overlap, creating a resonant effect that amplifies reproductive function disruptions. An individualized approach is essential to assess and address these interactions.

Did You Know?

- *The average age of menarche has dropped significantly over the last century, with most girls starting their periods by age 13.8.*
- *Stress, environmental pollutants, and energy imbalances contribute to irregular menstrual cycles in adolescents.*

Menstrual Cycle Disorders

How can we differentiate normal pubertal processes and the establishment of menstrual cycles from actual disorders? This question becomes critical when irregular cycles are typical in adolescents. When should we become concerned and seek medical evaluation to avoid overlooking potential health issues?

The most common concerns among parents and girls include persistent irregular cycles, heavy bleeding (menorrhagia), and painful periods (dysmenorrhea). While the primary factors influencing menstrual cycle regularity have been discussed, additional factors can disrupt the cycle. If these factors are present, they likely contribute to the problem. Until they are resolved or their impact is reduced, the cycle irregularities will persist. The biggest mistakes in such cases are misdiagnosis and unjustified treatment.

Menstrual cycle regulation involves a complex interaction between the brain (the control center) and the uterus (the target organ). This system, known as the hypothalamic-pituitary-ovarian axis, starts functioning cyclically with the increase in gonadotropins and the onset of menstruation.

The cycle begins with the maturation of follicles in the ovaries under the influence of pituitary gonadotropins. As follicles mature, they produce estrogens, which stimulate the growth of the uterine lining (endometrium). If ovulation occurs, the ruptured follicle transforms into the corpus luteum, producing progesterone. Progesterone inhibits further endometrial growth and prepares the uterus to receive a fertilized egg. If conception does not occur, levels of progesterone and estrogen drop significantly, leading to the shedding of the endometrium as menstruation.

Menstruation is a hormone withdrawal bleed triggered by the lowest levels of estrogen and progesterone.

These low hormone levels simultaneously signal the hypothalamus to release specific hormones that stimulate the pituitary gland. The pituitary, in turn, produces gonadotropins, initiating another cycle. This cyclicity is key to normal menstrual function.

While gonadotropins and sex hormones are the primary regulators of the menstrual cycle, numerous other substances are involved in egg maturation and cycle maintenance. Thousands of these substances exist, many with roles not yet fully understood. Disruptions at any level of this regulatory system, whether in the hypothalamus, pituitary gland, ovaries, or uterus, can lead to temporary or prolonged menstrual cycle irregularities.

Understanding these processes' complexity is essential to effectively identifying and managing menstrual disorders.

How to Identify Menstrual Cycle Disorders

If regular 28-30-day cycles are uncommon among adolescents, how can we differentiate normal cycle development from actual disorders? Although it is unhelpful to compare adolescent menstrual cycles to those of adult women, understanding norms and deviations is essential for identifying potential issues.

In terms of cycle length, menstrual cycles can be either too long or too short. Cycles longer than 40-45 days or shorter than 14-21 days may raise concerns. Long cycles are often associated with the absence of egg maturation and anovulation, typically regular during adolescence. This is generally categorized as a disruption of the first phase of the cycle, resulting in the absence of the second phase and a monophasic (anovulatory) cycle. Even during ovulation, adolescents often experience longer follicular phases than adult women. As girls mature, this phase shortens, leading to shorter cycles. Long menstrual cycles are, therefore, common among teenage girls.

Short cycles, by contrast, are typically associated with disruptions in the second phase, often linked to progesterone deficiency. However, it is essential to note that luteal phase deficiency in adolescents is rare and is primarily caused by issues with corpus luteum function or progesterone absorption by reproductive organs.

For adult women, having at least nine menstrual cycles per year is considered normal. Six to eight cycles annually may be sufficient for adolescents in the first three years of cycle establishment. If cycles are shorter than 21 days, resulting in as many as 16-17 cycles per year, this is unusual for teenage girls and warrants attention.

The primary cause of irregular cycles in adolescents is the immaturity of the regulatory mechanisms that govern menstruation, leading to a lack of consistent ovulation. Stress often exacerbates this situation. Anovulatory cycles occur in 55-82% of cases in the first two years following menarche. Over the next 1-2 years, this rate drops to about 50%, and within 2-3 additional years (five years after menarche), anovulatory cycles decrease to 10-20%. Parents should understand that if a girl begins menstruating at 13-14 years old, her cycles may remain irregular until she is 18-20. Factors such as physical and emotional stress or a low weight-to-height ratio can further delay the establishment of regular cycles. It is crucial for parents, especially mothers, to internalize this information to support their daughters better.

Changes in cycle length are not the only potential deviations; changes like menstruation may also occur. Periods may be very light, short, or heavy and prolonged. Girls and women often pay less attention to light periods than to heavy ones, as the latter cause more discomfort and concern.

Normal menstruation lasts up to seven days and sometimes up to ten days (with minimal bleeding during the last few days). Adolescents typically use 3-5 sanitary pads or tampons daily, depending on pad thickness and personal preferences. However, if pads need to be changed every 1-2 hours for the period, a medical evaluation is necessary.

Abnormal bleeding that occurs outside the normal menstrual cycle is classified as **abnormal uterine bleeding (AUB)** or, in some contexts, **juvenile uterine bleeding,** emphasizing its association with adolescence. It is essential to distinguish between AUB and heavy menstrual bleeding (HMB), now recognized as a separate diagnosis in modern gynecology.

AUB has various subtypes, with prevalence depending on the individual's age group. Among adolescents, the most common type is **dysfunctional uterine bleeding (DUB),** primarily linked to an immature reproductive system. Within this category, **hypothalamic bleeding** is the most frequent, highlighting the connection between the hypothalamus and ovarian regulation via the hypothalamic-pituitary-ovarian axis, which is still developing in adolescents.

In most cases, juvenile bleeding is not due to severe hormonal disorders or uterine diseases but stems from the ongoing maturation of the ovulation and menstruation processes. Observation and patience are often the best approaches, as these mechanisms need time to develop.

Further discussion of these deviations will continue throughout the book.

Did You Know?

- *Menstrual cycles in adolescents often remain irregular for several years, with up to 82% of cycles being anovulatory during the first two years after menarche.*
- *Abnormal uterine bleeding (AUB) in teenagers is typically linked to the immaturity of their reproductive system and rarely signals severe conditions.*

Uterine Bleeding in Adolescents

To characterize uterine bleeding, ranging from physiological (normal) to pathological, a standardized classification is used, often by doctors, to evaluate the nature of the bleeding:

Volume	**Regularity**	**Frequency**	**Duration**	**Other**
Heavy	Irregular	Frequent (4+ menstruations in 90 days or interval <24 days)	Prolonged (8+ days)	Intermenstrual
Normal	Regular	Normal	Normal	Premenstrual
Light	Absent (>90 days)	Rare (1-2 menstruations in 90 days or interval >38-45 days)	Short (<3 days)	Breakthrough

Premature menstruation, occurring before age 9, is another category within this framework. Abnormal uterine bleeding (AUB) may be classified as **acute** (sudden onset) or **chronic** (persisting for over six cycles).

While the table above provides a practical framework for assessing uterine bleeding, each girl or young woman must be evaluated individually, considering not only the nature of the bleeding but also her medical history, life circumstances, and factors affecting her menstrual cycle, as discussed in this book.

Adolescents, mainly, may experience heavy menstrual bleeding, often following prolonged absence of menstruation. This is typically because of estrogen without the balancing influence of progesterone, as ovulation and corpus luteum formation are often absent in this age group. Without progesterone, a condition known as **endometrial hyperplasia**, excessive growth of the uterine lining can occur. It's important to note that endometrial hyperplasia in adolescents is usually not pathological, and invasive interventions such as uterine cavity scraping are rarely necessary.

The detachment of hyperplastic endometrium can result in significant bleeding, regardless of the menstrual cycle day, or lead to heavy menstrual periods. However, other conditions must also be considered as potential causes of such bleeding.

In adolescent girls, the causes of heavy menstrual bleeding and AUB often differ from those in adult women. For adult women, common causes include growths such as polyps, fibroids, adenomyosis, malignant processes, hyperplasia, and, occasionally, other diseases.

In adolescents, **dysfunctional uterine bleeding (DUB)** due to anovulation is the most frequent cause. Blood disorders, specifically **coagulopathies** (blood clotting disorders), account for 7-48% of cases, depending on the source. Around 20% of cases are attributed to the inappropriate or unjustified use of hormonal medications or other drugs, such as anticoagulants, antipsychotics, or spironolactone, which can affect ovarian function, the uterus, and blood clotting. Additionally, nearly 20% of cases remain unexplained.

Understanding these distinctions is crucial for accurate diagnosis and appropriate management, particularly during the sensitive period of adolescence.

When to Pay Attention to Uterine Bleeding

- Menstrual cycles are irregular, occurring more frequently than every 21 days or less frequently than every 45 days (in the first year after menarche, cycles up to 45 days or slightly longer are considered normal).
- Bleeding persists for more than 7 days.
- A sanitary pad or tampon becomes saturated within 1 hour (normal usage is 3–6 pads or tampons per day).

- Blood clots larger than 2.5 cm are present in the discharge (it can be challenging to distinguish endometrial tissue from blood clots).
- Clothing and bedding become soaked due to heavy bleeding.

Acute bleeding episodes are the most common, but some adolescents experience chronic bleeding, recurring in every cycle. Chronic bleeding can significantly impact their quality of life, with nearly half of affected adolescents missing school during their periods and being unable to participate in physical, social, or extracurricular activities.

Key Steps in Providing Timely and Proper Care for an Adolescent with Uterine Bleeding

1. **Ensure the bleeding is not life-threatening**: Assess whether the adolescent is hemodynamically stable, meaning there is no immediate threat to life due to blood loss. This is the priority in managing such cases.
2. **Identify the bleeding source**: Determine whether the bleeding originates from external genitalia, the vagina, or the uterus. For example, trauma to the genital area could be the cause, requiring a thorough history and examination to identify the source accurately.
3. **Determine the cause of uterine bleeding**: In about 20% of cases, the exact cause remains unknown. However, identifying potential contributing factors such as hormonal imbalances, blood disorders, or medications is essential for effective management.
4. **Ascertain whether the bleeding is associated with an ovulatory or anovulatory cycle**:
    - Anovulatory cycles typically do not cause premenstrual or menstrual symptoms like pain or breast tenderness.
    - Ultrasound may not always detect the corpus luteum at the beginning of menstrual bleeding because it

shrinks significantly and can resemble other aging follicles.

Recognizing these signs and taking appropriate action can prevent complications, improve the adolescent's quality of life, and ensure proper reproductive health care.

Assessing Uterine Bleeding in Adolescents

A comprehensive evaluation of uterine bleeding in adolescents involves several steps to determine the underlying cause and ensure appropriate management. This assessment includes:

- **Overall Health Evaluation**: Examine the adolescent's general health and identify signs of anemia, such as fatigue, pale skin, or rapid heartbeat.
- **Family History Review**: Investigate any family history of bleeding disorders or other blood-related diseases that may predispose the child to abnormal bleeding.
- **Medication Review**: Evaluate the adolescent's medications, particularly those that could impact blood clotting, such as anticoagulants or certain hormonal treatments.
- **Pregnancy Testing**: Given that 60–70% of adolescents under 18 are sexually active, ruling out pregnancy is an essential part of the evaluation.
- **Infection and Injury Assessment**: Check for genital infections or injuries that could contribute to abnormal bleeding.
- **Thyroid Function Testing**: Thyroid dysfunction, particularly hypothyroidism, is a common cause of heavy menstrual bleeding. Studies show that 50–80% of adolescents with thyroid hypofunction experience excessive bleeding.
- **Blood Clotting Tests**: Screening for coagulopathies is critical, as blood disorders rank as the second most common cause of abnormal uterine bleeding in adolescents. However, only about 35% of girls are tested for these

conditions. Undiagnosed blood clotting disorders can manifest later in life during significant events like childbirth, surgery, or more severe bleeding episodes.

- **Systemic Disease Evaluation**: Systemic illnesses such as hepatitis, diabetes, kidney disease, and lupus can influence menstrual cycles and contribute to abnormal bleeding. These conditions should be considered as part of the diagnostic process.

In practice, identifying the exact cause of uterine bleeding in adolescents often requires multiple visits and a detailed, thorough investigation. Many countries have established guidelines for pediatricians and adolescent gynecologists to manage menstrual irregularities and abnormal bleeding. However, gaps in screening remain, particularly for coagulopathies, leaving some conditions undiagnosed until later in life.

A methodical approach that considers all potential influences on the menstrual cycle ensures the best outcomes for adolescents experiencing abnormal uterine bleeding.

Did You Know?

- *Heavy menstrual bleeding in adolescents is often linked to anovulation, where the absence of ovulation leads to imbalanced hormone levels.*
- *Undiagnosed blood clotting disorders contribute to up to 48% of abnormal uterine bleeding cases in adolescents, yet only about 35% are screened for these conditions.*

Heavy Menstrual Bleeding

Since adolescent cycles are often irregular, accurately assessing the situation and making a correct diagnosis can be challenging. Any heavy bleeding raises several questions for parents, the adolescent, and the doctor alike: Is it the result of a prolonged cycle with endometrial hyperplasia? Is it consistent with heavy menstruation with a standard endometrial thickness? Is it due to a blood clotting disorder? Unlike adult women, normal processes in adolescent girls can easily be mistaken for abnormalities, and actual abnormalities may go unnoticed. The age ranges from 11.5-12 to 21-22 are a "gray zone" in a young woman's life, where careful assessment, a gentle approach, patience, and restraint are needed, rather than hasty, aggressive interventions.

Continuing with the topic of bleeding, let's focus more on menstruation. As mentioned earlier, girls and women are less likely to complain about light periods than heavy ones, as it's much easier to manage with fewer pads or tampons without worrying about leakage or feeling significant moisture. While the bleeding may not always be objectively heavy, gynecology follows an unwritten rule: menstrual bleeding is considered heavy (excessive) when it feels heavy to the woman. And it's hard to disagree with this; if a woman feels discomfort due to "heavy" bleeding, she is likely to seek medical assistance.

In such cases, it is essential to determine whether the amount of bleeding is truly excessive or if it is an exaggerated subjective perception. Assessing the situation requires time and cannot be rushed. It is not appropriate for a girl or woman to receive an extensive list of tests and prescriptions immediately after visiting a doctor without a proper evaluation. Instead, the approach should begin with measures that do not require significant effort, energy, or financial expense.

When heavy menstrual bleeding is suspected, the girl may be advised to keep a specialized bleeding assessment chart. This chart tracks the number and type of pads or tampons used daily, their replacement frequency, and the child's overall condition.

A **menstrual diary** is also increasingly popular for evaluating menstrual bleeding. This diary includes information about:

- The use of medications (name, dose, and frequency of administration).
- Symptoms (e.g., pain, dizziness, weakness).
- Other essential details include missed school days due to poor general health.

Day	Day 1	Day 2	Day 3	Day 4	Day 5	Day 6	Day 7	Day 8
Thin (mini) pads	//				//	/		
Medium (regular) pads	/	///	//	///	//			
Thick (maxi/night) pads		/	///	//				
Blood clots			/					
Leakage			/					

By systematically tracking this information, evaluating the severity of bleeding becomes easier, as does determining whether further medical intervention is necessary.

Evaluating menstrual flow is inherently subjective. Research indicates that many women misinterpret the severity of their menstruation, with some perceiving light bleeding as heavy and others viewing genuinely heavy periods as normal and unproblematic.

Various methods have been attempted to quantify menstrual blood loss, but most have proven ineffective, expensive, or impractical (e.g., the alkaline hematin test). Counting the number of tampons or pads used is a common, imperfect approach. A tampon is estimated to absorb around 5 ml of blood, while sanitary pads can absorb 5-10 ml, depending on their type. However, pads vary widely, from thin daily liners to thick overnight pads, and most girls and women change them before they are fully saturated. In such cases, the presence of blood clots in the discharge often raises more concern than the pad or tampon absorption level.

Heavy menstrual bleeding is defined as excessive blood loss during menstruation that significantly impacts a girl's (or woman's) physical, emotional, and social quality of life. This bleeding may be accompanied by other symptoms or occur independently.

Up to 30% of adolescents report experiencing heavy menstrual bleeding, though only about 12% require hospitalization or intensive medical intervention.

Diagnosing heavy menstrual bleeding in adolescents follows a similar process as evaluating any bleeding, but the age at onset is a critical factor.

- ❖ If periods are excessively heavy from the start (from menarche), a **blood clotting disorder** should be suspected. Supporting clues include a family history of similar issues (e.g., the mother had heavy periods), cycle regularity, unexplained bruising, or subcutaneous bleeding.
- ❖ If menstruation was initially light or regular for the first 2-3 years but later became heavy or irregular, a **hormonal disorder** may be the cause.

Polycystic Ovary Syndrome (PCOS) is one potential diagnosis, particularly in adolescents, though it has become overdiagnosed in some countries due to the high costs of testing and treatment. To confirm PCOS, other indicators should also be present, such as obesity, excessive hair growth (hirsutism), and the absence of symptoms related to other bleeding disorders.

An accurate evaluation of menstrual health in adolescents requires a holistic approach, considering physical symptoms and the broader context of family history, hormonal patterns, and overall health.

Treating uterine bleeding in adolescents requires a carefully individualized approach rather than resorting to hormonal contraceptives or invasive procedures like uterine cavity scraping as quick solutions. In cases of acute anemia, hospitalization may be necessary, and treatment could involve blood transfusions, blood products, or hemostatic medications.

For **acute bleeding**, hormonal therapies, including combined oral contraceptives (COCs), progestins, or estrogens, are often prescribed. Bed rest is also recommended for adolescents with severe anemia and general weakness to aid recovery.

The use of **intravenous estrogen** to halt bleeding was first introduced in 1982, showing a 75% success rate by constricting endometrial blood vessels, stimulating endometrial growth, and enhancing clot formation. While estrogen is rarely used alone today, it is often combined with progesterone and administered in tablet form. COCs remain a preferred option for managing acute bleeding. Still, they are typically reserved for specific cases in adolescents due to concerns about long-term effects on their still-maturing hormonal regulation systems.

There is ongoing debate regarding the prolonged use of hormonal contraceptives (over months or years) for adolescents with heavy menstrual bleeding. Current guidelines lack clarity on which contraceptives to use, the optimal duration of therapy, and the long-term safety of COC use in adolescents whose cycle regulation mechanisms are not yet fully developed.

In recent years, synthetic progestins have become a popular alternative. These are commonly administered as mini-pill tablets, though the intrauterine hormonal system (e.g., Mirena) is sometimes used. However, the latter is rarely recommended for adolescents who are not sexually active.

Nonsteroidal anti-inflammatory drugs (NSAIDs), such as ibuprofen, are commonly prescribed when menstrual bleeding is accompanied by pain. They have proven effective in treating heavy menstrual bleeding, with mefenamic acid being particularly popular for this purpose.

Medications that affect blood clotting are tailored to the specific type of coagulopathy diagnosed. Antifibrinolytics and synthetic vasopressin analogs are among the most commonly used drugs in such cases.

More than 90% of adolescents with uterine bleeding respond well to hormonal and non-hormonal therapies, making surgical intervention rare. Surgical procedures, such as uterine cavity scraping, are avoided whenever possible, especially in adolescents with blood clotting disorders, as they can worsen the bleeding.

Modern medicine offers a variety of effective treatments for managing uterine bleeding. However, given that adolescents are still in the process of physical and hormonal development, the selection of medications must be cautious, deliberate, and thoroughly justified.

Did You Know?

- *Up to 30% of adolescents experience heavy menstrual bleeding, but only about 12% require intensive medical intervention or hospitalization.*
- *Heavy menstrual bleeding can be an early sign of blood clotting disorders, especially if it starts from menarche and is accompanied by unexplained bruising or a family history of similar issues.*

Hormonal Balance and Its Disruptions

Throughout this book, we've often discussed how hormonal balance shifts from birth through puberty. Elevated levels of male sex hormones are standard during adolescence, yet this frequently leads to misdiagnoses and unnecessary treatments.

What concerns adolescent girls most when their hormones start to "act up"? Their appearance. Skin issues like pimples, acne, and unwanted hair growth often dominate their worries. Teenagers rarely confide in their mothers or ask if they experienced similar changes. Was her skin also oily and acne-prone? Did she notice hair on her legs, or a few strands on her nipples, or, heaven forbid, above her upper lip? Many adolescents overlook their ethnic background and fail to observe similarities in their sisters, aunts, or grandmothers. Instead, they often focus on concealing these perceived "flaws" of feminine beauty.

What often happens next? If, along with these appearance concerns, a girl has irregular menstrual cycles, she may receive an immediate diagnosis of polycystic ovary syndrome (PCOS) at her first doctor's visit. Frequently, this leads to a prescription for an older hormonal contraceptive like "Diane-35" or a similar medication.

If the girl's mother experienced similar issues and followed this medical route, she would likely trust the doctor without questioning the diagnosis. Factors such as the child's underweight status, normal hormone levels (with only minor elevations in male hormones), and the transient nature of these symptoms often go unnoticed by the girl, her doctor, and her mother.

The result is a cycle of unnecessary treatment, often without addressing the root of the problem, and little understanding of the natural hormonal fluctuations during adolescence.

The Model Syndrome

You won't find "model syndrome" in any medical textbook or popular literature on women's health. This term originated in my publications, and it will eventually gain recognition among my colleagues.

What do modern adolescent girls and young women aspire to? To look like models. The omnipresence of advertisements showcasing teenage-like models feeds this desire. These models often resemble adolescents — thin, tall, "flat," pale, with an innocent expression that projects an air of purity.

Compare the models of the 1950s–70s with today's: the earlier figures, with their rounded shapes, curvier figures, and doll-like makeup, would be dismissed as "overweight" by current standards. Half a century ago, models and actresses didn't typically remove hair from their legs or bikini areas, a notion that would likely provoke a collective "ugh" from today's women and girls.

Adolescents today face relentless pressure from the media and entertainment industries to conform to the "modern woman" image.

Teenagers consume little written material but are immersed in visual and auditory input: phones and gadgets are their constant companions, delivering music, videos, and celebrity images, their icons of beauty and success. The ideal has shifted to a tall, slim woman who exudes independence and success and is surrounded by equally polished "cover-model" men. This figure is far from the athletic ideal of the past; in fact, sports participation among girls and women has been steadily declining. Instead, the "model" physique is often pursued through under-eating, fasting, and extreme dieting.

In the context of sexual immaturity and low body weight, menstrual irregularity or even absence is not pathological — it is, instead, a norm of "model syndrome." However, this "model" will likely end up at the doctor's office, often with her mother, who is more concerned about her daughter's irregular cycles than the girl herself.

The doctor typically orders lab tests, which reveal normal or slightly elevated levels of male hormones. Free testosterone is rarely measured, and mildly elevated cortisol or 17-OHP levels, both stress markers, might be flagged as abnormalities. The emotional intensity and categorically "nervous" nature of adolescents are often ignored, even though these factors naturally elevate stress-related hormones.

An ultrasound is often part of this scenario. The specialist might note *multifollicular* ovaries and a small uterus. If the doctor refrains from diagnosing "uterine hypoplasia" and prescribing hormones to "grow" the uterus, they may still focus on the multifollicular ovaries. The critical fact that most adolescents have anovulatory cycles, lacking a dominant follicle, is overlooked. Consequently, the uniform peripheral follicles, typical of this age group, are misinterpreted.

Another red flag for doctors is ovarian cysts, a topic we'll explore in another chapter.

Does all of this mean that these adolescents should be diagnosed with polycystic ovary syndrome (PCOS)? Not. Modern international guidelines advise against diagnosing PCOS before the age of 16. A thorough evaluation, including family history, is essential, for instance, considering if the mother has the condition. I continue to emphasize that in the majority of cases, these girls are not dealing with hormonal disorders. Instead, they are grappling with societal pressures and the unrealistic ideals encapsulated in what I call "model syndrome."

Ovarian Dysfunction or Hormonal Imbalance

What do adult women often hear from doctors when they seek help for menstrual cycle irregularities? Often, without a thorough investigation into whether the issue is new or recurring and without proper examination, they're quickly diagnosed with "ovarian dysfunction." Adolescent girls seeking medical advice for similar concerns frequently receive the same ambiguous label.

The term **"ovarian dysfunction"** is as non-specific and vague as "headache" or "birth injury" — a catch-all phrase used when the doctor prefers not to delve into a more precise diagnosis. "Dysfunction" means "impaired function."

So, what exactly is the function of the ovaries? They have two primary and interconnected roles:

1. To mature reproductive cells (egg cells or oocytes).
2. To produce hormones that support conception and overall reproductive health.

Without reproductive cell maturation, the ovaries are hormonally inactive or produce minimal hormones, as seen during menopause, pregnancy, or breastfeeding.

Similarly, the uterus cannot adequately prepare for pregnancy without follicle maturation. Thus, any disruption in the maturation of egg cells impairs ovarian function — the essence of "dysfunction."

A common synonym for "ovarian dysfunction" is **"hormonal imbalance,"** which is also not an accurate diagnosis. When this term appears in medical records, it signals diagnostic imprecision.

The female body, including that of adolescents, produces over 50 hormonally active substances. Some directly influence the ovaries by either stimulating or inhibiting their activity. Others act on different organs that, in turn, affect ovarian function, indirectly causing menstrual irregularities. As such, "hormonal imbalance" is akin to saying, "You're not sleeping well because your sleep is poor." Interestingly, when hormone levels (e.g., FSH, LH, estrogen, progesterone, testosterone) are tested, they often fall within normal ranges, even in irregular cycles.

The key to differentiating between normal and abnormal lies in understanding that occasional irregularities, often due to spontaneous anovulation, don't cause significant hormonal disruptions because there hasn't been enough time for such changes. Egg maturation takes several months, with the final two weeks of maturation being most influenced by pituitary and hypothalamic hormones.

When negative factors trigger spontaneous anovulation, the hypothalamus-pituitary system is typically affected first, long before the ovaries respond. As a result, delayed menstruation often reflects a past adverse event—emotional, physical, or otherwise—that temporarily slowed or paused egg maturation. If the event is brief, the irregularity resolves quickly. If prolonged or intense, cycle disruptions may persist and could be accompanied by hormonal deviations.

It's crucial to understand that ovarian dysfunction is usually "triggered from above" — the root cause often lies in the regulatory system that governs ovarian function. Direct ovarian impairment at the organ level is far less common and usually results from congenital underdevelopment or damage, such as surgical removal of ovarian tissue. A significant loss of follicular apparatus leads to ovarian dysfunction, which directly affects hormone production.

If the ovaries are normal in size and no functional cysts are detected that could disrupt the cycle, the underlying cause likely lies outside the ovaries. Identifying such causes often requires 3–6 months of observation and repeated hormone assessments, which can be financially and logistically challenging for families.

Despite this, many doctors continue to record "ovarian dysfunction" as the sole diagnosis in medical records, frequently prescribing hormonal contraceptives as the standard treatment, sometimes for several months or even a year.

Both parents and adolescents need to understand that "ovarian dysfunction" is not a diagnosis. Instead, it describes a menstrual irregularity that can arise from numerous underlying causes. If hormone levels are normal, the focus should shift to evaluating weight, psycho-emotional health, nutrition, rest patterns, and other potential health factors.

Did You Know?

- *Most adolescents with irregular menstrual cycles do not have a hormonal disorder; these irregularities are often part of normal pubertal development. Diagnosing conditions like PCOS before the age of 16 is generally discouraged.*
- *"Ovarian dysfunction" and "hormonal imbalance" are not specific diagnoses but rather broad terms indicating menstrual irregularities often caused by factors outside the ovaries, such as stress or weight changes.*

A Few Words About Male Sex Hormones

I've written and spoken extensively about male sex hormones in recent years, primarily to dispel the myths and misconceptions surrounding them. One of the most persistent myths is the idea that male sex hormones are "enemies" of the female body simply because they are "male." However, a critical fact often overlooked — even by some doctors — is that **all female hormones are derived from male sex hormones.** In other words, without male hormones, female hormones could not exist.

Another lesser-known fact is that **the female body produces significantly more male sex hormones than female hormones**. Only a tiny fraction of these androgens is converted into estrogens, yet this small amount is sufficient to maintain essential female functions.

A third important point, often misunderstood, is that **of the five primary types of androgens, only testosterone and dihydrotestosterone (DHT) have true androgenic (male sex hormone) activity**. The other three, dehydroepiandrosterone (DHEA) and androstenedione, are precursors and metabolites without direct androgenic effects. Unfortunately, when testing an adolescent girl's hormones, there's often a focus on these precursors, even though they lack androgenic properties. Many doctors aren't aware of which specific hormones are relevant, leading to unnecessary testing and misinterpreting results.

Another common mistake is initiating treatment for a minor elevation in a single hormone without considering symptoms or the hormone's actual function. For example, if the elevated hormone lacks androgenic properties, treating it is typically unnecessary and can lead to unwarranted interventions.

In the female body, testosterone exists in two forms: bound to proteins and free. **Only free testosterone is biologically active**. However, the units used to measure bound and free testosterone differ, which often confuses them. People frequently compare numbers without paying attention to the measurement units, leading to misinterpretations and unnecessary worry.

Cortisol, produced by the adrenal glands, is another hormone commonly tested in menstrual irregularities, but it is not a male sex hormone. Cortisol is a stress hormone that rises rapidly in response to negative and positive stimuli, such as fear, stress, lack of sleep, physical exertion, or emotional excitement. Cortisol also breaks down more slowly than other stress hormones, allowing it to impact tissues and organs longer.

A byproduct of cortisol breakdown is 17-hydroxyprogesterone (17-OHP), another steroid hormone frequently measured in girls' blood or urine. Slightly elevated 17-OHP levels often lead to incorrect diagnoses of hyperandrogenism (excess male hormones) and subsequent unnecessary treatment. It's crucial to understand that 17-OHP is not an indicator of hyperandrogenism.

Female endocrinology, the study of women's hormonal balance, is a complex and specialized field. Unfortunately, it is often underemphasized in medical training, particularly regarding the biochemistry of hormone production, metabolism, and organ response. Many gynecologists lack a solid understanding of endocrinology, and endocrinologists often have limited expertise in gynecology. This gap leaves adolescent girls caught in a cycle of repeated testing and extended hormonal treatments that may not address their actual concerns.

To avoid such pitfalls, focusing on the individual's symptoms and overall health is vital rather than solely relying on numbers from laboratory results. Proper education and a nuanced understanding of female endocrinology are essential to prevent unnecessary interventions and support healthy development.

Hyperandrogenism

The term "hyperandrogenism" is frequently encountered in the medical evaluation of adolescent girls and young women. However, it is not a definitive diagnosis but rather a condition characterized by elevated levels of male hormones in a woman's body. As previously discussed, there are several types of male hormones, so identifying which specific hormones are elevated and understanding their impact on the body is crucial beyond just interpreting lab results.

One important rule in endocrinology is that **diagnoses should never rely on a single hormone test**, particularly in the absence of apparent symptoms of hyperandrogenism. Isolated elevations in hormone levels are often due to lab errors or physiological fluctuations.

Many everyday aspects of puberty are mistaken for signs of hyperandrogenism. The most common concerns include increased body hair in socially undesirable areas, menstrual irregularities, and frequent anovulation. During puberty, hair naturally appears in the underarms, bikini area, legs, around the nipples, and along the midline of the abdomen. Additionally, menstrual cycles often remain irregular in adolescents as the hypothalamic-pituitary-ovarian axis matures.

As girls mature, issues related to self-image often lead to attempts at extreme body modification through fasting, restrictive diets, or intense physical exercise. These practices can exacerbate cycle irregularities and stress the endocrine system.

Complaints of oily skin, acne, and brittle hair are also common. However, these are not necessarily indicative of hyperandrogenism. Many adolescents and parents lack education on proper skincare, leading to aggressive treatments with multiple ineffective products, further worsening skin issues.

True hyperandrogenism involves more serious symptoms, such as:

- Clitoromegaly (clitoral enlargement)
- Deepening of the voice
- Masculine skeletal development patterns

In adult women, hyperandrogenism can present as hirsutism (excessive hair growth), persistent acne, male-pattern hair loss, menstrual irregularities, infertility, and other metabolic disturbances.

These signs warrant medical attention when they appear suddenly, worsen over time, or cause discomfort for the individual. Androgens are produced by the ovaries, adrenal glands, and peripheral tissues (such as fat). Elevated male hormones can result from several mechanisms:

1. Increased testosterone production by the ovaries or adrenal glands, including hormone-secreting tumors.
2. Disruptions in testosterone binding to proteins lead to elevated free testosterone.
3. Metabolic issues with androgen breakdown and elimination, often due to genetic enzyme deficiencies.

Some conditions linked to hyperandrogenism include:

- Polycystic Ovary Syndrome (PCOS): A complex metabolic disorder involving elevated testosterone, high insulin levels, and often obesity.
- Congenital Adrenal Hyperplasia (CAH) is a hereditary condition caused by enzyme deficiencies, resulting in adrenal cortex hyperplasia and elevated androgen production (CAH has classic and non-classic forms, each with varying symptoms).
- Androgen-Secreting Tumors: Ovarian or adrenal tumors producing male hormones. These are rare but often malignant, with the potential to metastasize.

Mild to moderate increases in androgen levels are common in adolescents and often reflect normal hormonal fluctuations during puberty. These cases typically do not require extensive testing or aggressive treatment, especially if symptoms are absent or mild.

In cases of significant testosterone elevation, further evaluation is warranted to rule out severe conditions such as tumors or adrenal hyperplasia. However, treatment should never be based on a single hormone test. A holistic approach, considering the individual's symptoms, medical history, and physical examination, is essential for appropriate management.

Did You Know?

- *Female hormones, like estrogen, are synthesized from male sex hormones, specifically androgens. Without male hormones, the body cannot produce essential female hormones.*
- *Elevated testosterone levels in adolescent girls are often expected and linked to natural pubertal changes, not necessarily indicative of conditions like polycystic ovary syndrome (PCOS).*

Pimples and Acne

Almost every adolescent girl or young woman encounters pimples, most commonly on the face but also the back, shoulders, and chest. While not every pimple qualifies as "acne," this term specifically refers to an inflammatory process affecting hair follicles and sebaceous glands. Acne is characterized by an overgrowth of keratinocytes (skin cells) and increased oil production.

Up to 85% of teenagers experience acne, with around 20% seeking medical attention due to its significant emotional and physical impact. The presence of bacteria, particularly *Propionibacterium acnes*, often exacerbates the condition. Blackheads, or comedones, are another hallmark feature of acne.

Acne primarily occurs between the ages of 15 and 19, though its exact causes remain unclear. Elevated male hormones, common during puberty, are a significant trigger. However, adult women may also experience breakouts, often linked to stress, exhaustion, fasting, sleep deprivation, or wearing synthetic clothing.

Although acne affects many adolescents and some adults, clinical studies on it are relatively scarce, as it typically resolves naturally over time. For most girls, acne diminishes as their menstrual cycles become regular and they adopt consistent skincare routines. Explaining to adolescents that acne is often temporary and manageable through lifestyle changes and proper skin care can be reassuring and practical.

Acne diagnosis is straightforward in most cases and does not require extensive testing. Testing is only necessary in severe or resistant cases.

Proper skincare is critical for managing acne.

Many adolescents mistakenly believe that aggressively treating pimples with numerous products will speed up recovery. However, acne is a chronic condition linked to hormonal fluctuations, lifestyle factors, and stress responses. Overusing skincare products often worsens the problem.

- **Cleansing and Hygiene:**

Over-cleansing strips the skin of natural oils, prompting it to produce more oil, exacerbating acne. Gentle washing with lukewarm water and neutral soap every other day may suffice for maintaining healthy skin. Residual shampoo or conditioner on the skin after hair washing can also trigger acne, so it's essential to rinse the face thoroughly after showering.

- **Environmental Impact:**

Skin reacts to temperature fluctuations, such as moving between cold outdoor air and heated indoor environments. These changes can stimulate oil production as a protective mechanism. Over-cleansing can increase skin sensitivity and inflammation.

- **Emotional Support**

Psychological factors often play a significant role in acne. Emotional distress about skin appearance can create a vicious cycle that diminishes the effectiveness of other treatments. Though rarely considered, consulting a psychotherapist or counselor can be as impactful as medical interventions.

Medications and Alternative Treatments

The acne treatment market is vast, offering over-the-counter and prescription products. Medications include:

- **Topical Treatments:**

  These remain the first choice due to their effectiveness and minimal side effects.

- **Systemic Treatments:**

  Oral medications like synthetic vitamin A derivatives, antibiotics, steroids, hormonal therapies, and anti-androgens may be used in more severe cases. However, these require careful oversight.

- **Hormonal Contraceptives:**

  Certain new-generation progestins can improve skin conditions and may be prescribed if hormonal imbalances or contraceptive needs are present. However, hormonal treatments should not be the first-line approach for acne, especially in adolescents.

- **Alternative Therapies:**

  Laser treatments, light therapy, and photodynamic therapy are increasingly popular but remain controversial regarding their long-term effectiveness.

Concerns about the prolonged use of antibiotics can lead to resistance and the rationality of specific acne treatments. Because acne management often involves multiple professionals (dermatologists, cosmetologists, etc.), outcomes can be inconsistent if not carefully coordinated.

When managing acne in adolescents, avoid excessive testing or aggressive treatments, particularly self-medication. Instead, consult a specialist to recommend an individualized and balanced treatment plan. Adolescents should be educated about acne's natural progression and taught simple, effective skincare practices to manage the condition while maintaining emotional well-being.

Hirsutism

Pursuing "smooth skin," fueled by modern beauty standards, often leaves girls feeling frustrated and self-conscious about unwanted hair. Mothers who have faced similar struggles and adhere to beauty traditions may worry that their daughter's hair growth indicates a hormonal issue. Online information frequently attributes hirsutism to elevated male hormones, causing unnecessary anxiety.

Hereditary factors primarily determine hair growth, as hair follicles develop during embryonic development. Other influences include androgen levels, androgen metabolism, proteins that bind sex hormones, and the sensitivity of hair follicles to androgens. Skin infections like acne can increase hair sensitivity to these hormones.

There are two main types of hair:

- Vellus hair: Fine, short, unpigmented, and independent of androgen levels.
- Terminal hair: Coarser, longer, pigmented, and influenced by various hormones.

If a girl notices a light fuzz on her chin or cheeks, this is typically vellus hair and not a sign of illness.

Hirsutism refers to the excessive growth of terminal hair in a male-pattern distribution, often due to elevated male hormone levels. Common areas include:

- Upper lip
- Chin
- Cheeks (sideburns)
- Ears
- Back
- Chest
- Around the nipples

- Lower abdomen
- Pubic area
- Thighs

It's important to remember that some hair growth in these areas can be **expected**. A balanced assessment is crucial to distinguish between normal hair growth and hirsutism.

More concerning is **virilization**, which includes hirsutism along with other masculinizing signs, such as:

- Deepening of the voice
- Male-pattern muscle development
- Clitoral enlargement
- Balding at the temples

Virilization typically suggests high androgen levels caused by ovarian or adrenal tumors and is often accompanied by the cessation of menstruation.

Another condition, hypertrichosis, involves increased hair growth unrelated to male hormones. Hypertrichosis is often hereditary and constitutional, running in families, and may represent a normal variation rather than a health issue.

Sudden or progressive hirsutism may indicate hormonal imbalances, such as:

- Polycystic ovary syndrome (PCOS)
- Cushing's syndrome
- Congenital adrenal hyperplasia
- Androgen-producing tumors of the ovaries or adrenal glands

Sometimes, hirsutism arises from androgen production or metabolism issues without an identifiable disease. Medications that increase androgen levels can also contribute to hirsutism.

A detailed medical history and physical examination are essential to determining the cause of hirsutism. Doctors may recommend photographing affected areas to monitor treatment progress. Special scales, like the Ferriman-Gallwey scoring system, quantify the severity of hirsutism.

Laboratory tests are crucial for ruling out androgen-producing ovarian or adrenal tumors. These tests typically include:

- Free and total testosterone levels
- Dehydroepiandrosterone sulfate (DHEAS)
- Androstenedione
- 17-hydroxyprogesterone

Imaging studies (ultrasound, CT, or MRI) may be necessary if hormonal levels suggest a tumor or other underlying condition. Treatment depends on the underlying cause and the severity of hair growth. It's important to remember that hirsutism itself is not a disease but rather a symptom of potential hormonal imbalance.

Standard treatment options include:

1. **Medical Management**
    - **Hormonal treatments:** Oral contraceptives, anti-androgens (like spironolactone), and glucocorticoids (for congenital adrenal hyperplasia).
    - **Topical treatments:** Eflornithine cream can slow facial hair growth.
2. **Lifestyle Changes**
    - Weight management can reduce androgen levels in women with PCOS or obesity.
3. **Cosmetic Procedures**
    - **Laser hair removal** and **intense pulsed light (IPL):** Effective for reducing hair density over time.
    - **Electrolysis:** Offers permanent hair removal but can be time-consuming and expensive.
    - Waxing, shaving, or depilatory creams provide temporary relief.
4. **Psychological Support**
    - Emotional distress from hirsutism can significantly affect self-esteem, making psychological support or counseling a valuable part of treatment.

For most adolescents, hirsutism is constitutional or hereditary and often requires no treatment beyond cosmetic management. However, sudden or severe hair growth, virilization, or associated symptoms should prompt a comprehensive evaluation by a specialist. Parents and adolescents should understand that while hirsutism can be distressing, it is manageable with the right approach.

Did You Know?

- *Up to 85% of teenagers experience acne, with hormonal changes during puberty being a significant trigger, though it often resolves naturally as cycles regularize.*
- *Hirsutism, or excess hair growth in areas where men typically have hair, can sometimes indicate hormonal imbalances but is often hereditary and not linked to a disease.*

Polycystic Ovary Syndrome (PCOS)

Over the past decade, polycystic ovary syndrome (PCOS) has shifted from being a little-known and rare condition to a widely discussed diagnosis, often misapplied to adolescent girls and young women, particularly in countries lacking clear diagnostic and treatment protocols. This rise in diagnoses has also made PCOS a "profitable" condition, involving extensive testing, long-term treatments, and reliance on hormonal medications and frequent medical consultations.

For many adolescent girls, PCOS is an unfamiliar term. However, concerned mothers, worried about their daughters' irregular menstrual cycles, often reflecting on their own past experiences, frequently initiate medical visits that lead to discussions about this "intimidating" diagnosis.

PCOS is a condition affecting women of reproductive age, characterized by symptoms like irregular menstrual cycles and the potential presence of multiple small ovarian cysts (follicles). Historically, it was known as **Stein-Leventhal syndrome.** Prevalence estimates suggest PCOS affects 5-10% of women from adolescence to menopause. However, differences in diagnostic approaches, particularly between Europe and the United States, contribute to confusion and misdiagnoses.

In Europe, PCOS is often diagnosed based on a single ultrasound finding of polycystic ovaries, even though 20-25% of all women naturally have polycystic ovaries, especially during adolescence. At this age, cycle irregularities and anovulatory cycles are typical, making polycystic ovaries a normal physiological finding rather than an indicator of disease. Other conditions, such as elevated prolactin levels, adrenal androgen excess, bulimia, or anorexia, can also cause similar ovarian appearances.

In contrast, American guidelines do not consider ultrasound findings alone sufficient for diagnosing PCOS. Instead, they emphasize a combination of clinical symptoms, laboratory results, and imaging. This discrepancy often leads to false-positive or false-negative diagnoses, further complicating the condition's management.

PCOS is an **endocrine-metabolic disorder** affecting hormonal balance, metabolism, and ovarian function. It involves disruptions in the hypothalamic-pituitary-ovarian axis and irregular gonadotropin production, which overstimulate the ovaries. Typical symptoms include:

- Irregular menstrual cycles (oligomenorrhea or amenorrhea)
- Anovulation (lack of egg maturation)
- Hyperandrogenism (elevated male hormone levels, causing acne or excessive hair growth)
- Obesity (present in 75% of cases, with moderate obesity in 50% of patients)

Laboratory findings often show elevated luteinizing hormone (LH), male hormones (testosterone), insulin (hyperinsulinemia), and lipids (hyperlipidemia).

Adolescents are frequently misdiagnosed with PCOS due to normal developmental variations mistaken for pathological signs. Let's explore two common concerns:

1. Oligomenorrhea in Adolescents

Oligomenorrhea refers to menstrual cycles longer than 35 days, but this definition applies mainly to adult women. In adolescents, prolonged cycles are often regular as their hypothalamic-pituitary-ovarian axis matures. Key statistics:

- In the first year post-menarche, 75% of cycles last 21-45 days.
- Even two years later, 85% of cycles remain within this range.
- Five years after menarche, 95% of cycles are 21-40 days long, and 75% are ovulatory.

Cycles may remain irregular until age 18-20, mainly if stress, low body weight, or other external factors are present.

2. Hyperandrogenism

Hyperandrogenism is another frequently misinterpreted PCOS indicator. Adolescents naturally experience elevated male hormone levels and insulin resistance during puberty. However, androgen norms for this age group remain undefined, leading to confusion. acne, mild hair growth, and irregular cycles are common in adolescence but do not necessarily indicate PCOS. Diagnostic criteria for hyperandrogenism in adults should not be applied to adolescents.

Some experts argue for renaming PCOS as "Metabolic Syndrome" since metabolic disruptions, not polycystic ovaries, are the primary issue. Adolescents with metabolic syndrome markers (e.g., insulin resistance and obesity) are more likely to develop PCOS later in life. For underweight girls, irregular cycles and anovulation are rarely linked to PCOS.

Polycystic ovary syndrome (PCOS) is not merely a reproductive disorder but a multifaceted condition with significant implications for metabolic and long-term health. Beyond irregular menstrual cycles and infertility, PCOS increases the risk of developing type 2 diabetes, cardiovascular disease, and endometrial cancer. Chronic low-grade inflammation and insulin resistance, hallmark features of PCOS, exacerbate these risks. Early diagnosis and lifestyle interventions, including tailored dietary and exercise programs, can mitigate these complications. Incorporating these perspectives ensures a holistic understanding of PCOS, empowering patients to manage their condition proactively.

Treatment strategies depend on age, symptoms, and individual priorities. Adolescents may prioritize managing acne and hair growth, while adults may focus on regulating cycles or addressing infertility. Key approaches include:

1. Weight Management

For women with obesity, gradual weight loss often reduces androgen and insulin levels, improving symptoms. Extreme dieting or rapid weight loss can exacerbate menstrual irregularities, so moderate, sustainable weight loss is recommended for adolescents.

2. Hormonal Contraceptives

Oral contraceptives (OCs) are commonly prescribed to regulate cycles and manage symptoms like acne or hirsutism. However, high-dose contraceptives are inappropriate for adolescents. Hormonal therapy suppresses ovulation rather than restoring it and is not a first-line treatment for young girls.

3. Metformin

The antidiabetic drug metformin is occasionally used for insulin resistance in PCOS but is rarely recommended for adolescents due to limited evidence of efficacy.

4. Avoiding Surgical Interventions

Surgical treatments, such as ovarian drilling, are generally unsuitable for adolescents, as they deplete the ovarian follicular reserve, risking infertility and early menopause.

Parents and healthcare providers must approach PCOS cautiously in adolescents. Overdiagnosis and premature treatment with hormones or surgery can harm a young girl's developing hypothalamic-pituitary-ovarian axis. Careful monitoring and addressing underlying factors like diet, weight, and emotional well-being are critical. Diagnosis should be reserved for cases meeting well-defined criteria, avoiding unnecessary interventions in the absence of clear evidence of PCOS.

Did You Know?

- *Polycystic ovary syndrome (PCOS) is one of the most overdiagnosed conditions in adolescent girls, with up to 20-25% of all young women having polycystic ovaries on ultrasound. This finding is normal during adolescence.*
- *Early lifestyle interventions, including balanced nutrition and regular physical activity, can significantly reduce the long-term risks associated with PCOS, such as type 2 diabetes and cardiovascular disease.*

Lower Abdominal Pain

Lower abdominal pain is a common experience in almost every woman's life, yet everyone uniquely perceives it. Many women immediately seek help from a gynecologist, assuming that any discomfort "down there" must be related to a gynecological issue. This misconception that lower abdominal pain is always linked to reproductive organs persists and is often passed down from mothers to daughters. The concern is not merely the presence of pain but the tendency to leave a gynecologist's office with a diagnosis, whether accurate or not. Unfortunately, this cycle perpetuates fear and misunderstanding as women unknowingly transfer their anxieties to their daughters, who often repeat the same pattern.

The pelvic area, where the reproductive organs are located, is tightly packed. It also contains other critical structures, including the intestines, urinary system, nerves, blood vessels, lymph nodes, ligaments, and muscles. These organs are closely arranged, with no empty spaces between them. Periodically, some organs may change in size or position, affecting neighboring structures like the intestines, bladder, or uterus, causing discomfort or pain in the lower abdomen.

In most cases, however, the source of the pain is **not gynecological**. Issues with the intestines, often due to an unhealthy diet, or bladder discomfort, such as irritation or infection, are frequent culprits. Despite this, girls, and sometimes their mothers, often seek help from a gynecologist, where non-gynecological causes like dietary habits or urinary health are sometimes overlooked.

Educating women and adolescents about the various potential causes of lower abdominal pain can help break this cycle of misunderstanding and encourage a more comprehensive approach to health.

Pain Perception and Assessment

Pain perception is inherently subjective and influenced by an individual's pain threshold. Some people endure intense pain stoically without complaint, while others may perceive even mild bloating as severe discomfort. This pain threshold is influenced by genetically modulated nervous system sensitivity, life experiences, and learned responses. In families where parents, especially mothers, frequently vocalize pain (sometimes to manipulate others), there is a high chance of daughters developing similar patterns of complaint and sensitivity toward pain.

Specific indicators can help gauge pain intensity, even if someone hardly complains. Pupil dilation, increased pulse and breathing rates, and elevated blood pressure can all signal pain, and they are often used to detect pain feigning. However, when the pain is mild, these indicators may not be present, which doesn't mean the person isn't experiencing pain.

Children's experiences and expressions of pain differ significantly from those of adults. Many children struggle to describe the nature or location of their pain accurately, and healthcare professionals often lack deep knowledge of assessing pediatric pain. Studies from North America show that in educational settings, veterinary colleges dedicate the most hours to pain assessment, followed by nursing schools, with medical schools spending the least time on the subject.

Various methods exist for evaluating pain in children, tailored to different age groups. For girls over 8, a ten-point pain scale is often practical, as most can count to ten at this age.

In medical evaluations, clinicians focus on distinguishing between episodic pain (random or infrequent occurrences) and cyclic pain (regular, often tied to menstrual cycles) and determining whether it is acute (sharp, sudden, intense) or chronic (persistent, usually mild and self-limiting).

An autonomous nervous system governs the pelvic organs, so signals from a diseased organ are sent to specific regions of the spinal cord that also receive signals from other organs.

Consequently, pain may radiate to the lower back, tailbone, or other pelvis areas, making pinpointing its exact source challenging and sometimes impossible.

Acute pelvic pain typically indicates an urgent issue, such as rupture, bleeding, perforation, or organ displacement. It's crucial to consider the pain's location, even if the affected organs aren't always immediately apparent. For example, pain in the upper abdomen might suggest issues with the esophagus, stomach, pancreas, liver, or gallbladder. Umbilical pain can indicate problems with the small intestine, appendix, upper ureter, or ovaries. In contrast, suprapubic pain is often associated with conditions of the lower intestines, bladder, lower ureters, or uterus. Shoulder pain accompanying abdominal pain suggests diaphragm injury.

Acute pain can manifest in various forms: intermittent, rhythmic, constant, sharp (like a knife), or dull, and may worsen with body movement. It can also be accompanied by chills, nausea, vomiting, vaginal bleeding, or even loss of consciousness.

Pelvic inflammatory disease (often previously labeled as inflammation of the ovaries or appendages) may cause persistent, acute pain lasting over two days. It's important to remember that pelvic organ inflammation usually results from sexually transmitted infections commonly observed in sexually active adolescents.

A child experiencing acute pain, regardless of age, should be hospitalized for evaluation, identification of the pain's cause, and urgent care.

When the reproductive system is inactive in young girls, pain usually originates from the intestines, often accompanied by constipation or diarrhea, or less frequently from urinary tract conditions (such as cystitis or pyelonephritis). Rarely pain arises from other causes.

In adolescence, cyclic pain is more common and generally physiological, signifying normal function, especially during menstruation (dysmenorrhea). Pain can also precede menstruation, known as premenstrual syndrome (PMS).

Dysmenorrhea and PMS typically occur with regular ovulation, indicating a normal hormonal profile.

Mid-cycle pain accompanied by slight bleeding, known as **Mittelschmerz**, results from ovulation. This discomfort arises from the peritoneal reaction to fluid released when a mature follicle ruptures, which is part of the ovulatory syndrome and is not considered pathological. Mittelschmerz generally lasts a few hours around ovulation.

Two other frequent gynecological conditions associated with chronic pelvic pain include endometriosis and congenital abnormalities of the reproductive system.

Did You Know?

- *Lower abdominal pain is not always gynecological in origin. It is often linked to non-reproductive organs, such as the intestines or bladder, emphasizing the need for a holistic approach to diagnosis and treatment.*
- *Pain perception varies widely among individuals and can be influenced by genetics, emotional state, and learned behaviors, making pain assessment highly subjective and unique to each person.*

Painful periods

Research indicates that painful menstruation affects 43-93% of adolescents, meaning nearly every girl may experience menstrual pain at least once, just as many adult women do. However, recurring painful episodes, known as dysmenorrhea or algodysmenorrhea, can disrupt a teenager's life and raise concerns.

The exact cause of menstrual pain remains unclear. It is believed that pain arises from uterine contractions. Although uterine contractions occur in all girls during menstruation and sometimes between cycles, some experience these contractions with accompanying lower abdominal pain.

Another factor contributing to painful periods is the buildup of specific substances - prostaglandins and arachidonic acid that trigger an inflammation-like response, irritate pain receptors in the pelvic organs, and increase uterine muscle contractions.

Progesterone-related tissue swelling in the uterus, including the muscle layer, may compress nerve endings, causing lower abdominal pain. There may also be other underlying causes.

Genetic factors might play a role in dysmenorrhea, as studies have found a familial link among over half of women and their female relatives who experience painful menstruation, possibly due to the production of certain factors.

Painful periods are often accompanied by heavier menstrual flow.

Primary dysmenorrhea, caused by natural uterine contractions, is found in about 50% of healthy women. Typically, the first episodes of dysmenorrhea begin in young girls and women two to three years after the onset of menstruation, once cycles become regular. Symptoms appear at the start of menstruation and usually last 32-48 hours. Among adolescents, 55% experience nausea, and 24% may have vomiting during painful periods.

Secondary dysmenorrhea is associated with specific reproductive system conditions and is rare in adolescents, except for cases involving intestinal or urinary tract issues. Dysmenorrhea is often a "diagnosis of exclusion," confirmed only after other causes of pelvic pain are ruled out. However, it can usually be diagnosed based on detailed questioning without extensive tests.

Most cases of dysmenorrhea do not require treatment, as the pain is typically manageable. However, in 21% of adolescents with painful periods, symptoms are severe, with nearly 30% unable to attend school or carry out daily activities.

Various treatment options exist, both medicinal and alternative. The primary goals are to reduce prostaglandin levels in the uterine tissues and shorten the duration of menstruation. Treatment choice depends on other reproductive conditions and the girl's preferences. Dysmenorrhea treatment is typically cyclical, requiring at least 3-5 cycles to show improvement, with some cases needing longer courses.

Traditional treatment for dysmenorrhea includes nonsteroidal anti-inflammatory drugs (NSAIDs) like ibuprofen, aspirin, naproxen, and mefenamic acid, which suppress prostaglandin production. For best results, NSAIDs should be taken 5-10 days before menstruation begins and during the first two days. COX-2 inhibitors and acetaminophen (Tylenol) also provide relief by reducing hormone levels. Though less effective than aspirin or ibuprofen, acetaminophen has fewer side effects.

If NSAIDs prove ineffective, combined hormonal contraceptives (pills, skin patches, or rarely vaginal rings) may be offered to suppress ovulation and reduce menstrual flow.

Dietary adjustments can alleviate symptoms. Starting from the second phase of the cycle (about 14 days before menstruation), a diet rich in whole grains, fresh vegetables, and fiber while reducing saturated fats and commercial drinks may help. Eating more fish and eggs and taking omega-3 supplements can also aid in managing menstrual pain. Limiting salt, caffeine, sugar, and alcohol intake before and during menstruation is often beneficial, as is avoiding intensive physical activity.

Alternative therapies like acupuncture, reflexology, yoga, meditation, and spinal massage may also reduce dysmenorrhea symptoms. A warm compress on the lower abdomen for two days, especially at bedtime, can significantly alleviate menstrual pain.

Pelvic Inflammatory Disease (PID)

Pelvic inflammatory disease (PID) primarily refers to the inflammation of the uterus, fallopian tubes, and, less commonly, the ovaries. Historically, terms like adnexitis, oophoritis, or salpingo-oophoritis were used to describe inflammation based on the affected reproductive organs. However, PID is most often caused by sexually transmitted infections (STIs) that predominantly affect the uterus and fallopian tubes, with ovarian involvement being rare.

PID presents a significant risk to reproductive health, particularly to the fallopian tubes. Inflammation can lead to scarring and damage, resulting in infertility. In rare and severe cases, PID may progress to peritonitis, a dangerous inflammation of the abdominal lining. While PID is exceptionally rare in young girls, its occurrence in this group should prompt serious concerns about possible sexual abuse. Conversely, in sexually active adolescents, PID is relatively common and warrants immediate attention.

Parents must understand that activities such as sitting on a cold surface or exposure to freezing temperatures do not cause inflammation of the ovaries, fallopian tubes, or uterus. These long-standing beliefs are myths. While cold exposure can increase the likelihood of bladder inflammation, particularly in children who frequently delay urination, this condition only causes discomfort in the pelvic area. It does not extend to other pelvic organs.

Symptoms of PID in adolescents often differ from those seen in adult women. For instance, vaginal discharge in young girls may appear different in color or consistency, making it challenging to distinguish between normal physiological discharge and pathological changes. However, increased discharge accompanied by other inflammatory signs may indicate PID.

In younger girls, PID may not always present with significant lower abdominal pain, though some discomfort might still occur. More frequently, symptoms include a noticeable rise in body temperature or fever, which may initially be mistaken for a common cold or unrelated illness. Nausea and vomiting are also frequent symptoms in PID cases.

For menstruating girls, PID can sometimes lead to intermenstrual spotting or bleeding, further complicating the diagnosis.

When PID is suspected, it is critical to rule out other conditions with overlapping symptoms, such as appendicitis or urinary system infections like pyelonephritis. The differentiation between these conditions is vital for accurate diagnosis and effective treatment.

Acute episodes of PID always necessitate hospitalization. Hospital care ensures proper diagnostic procedures and timely treatment initiation, which is crucial to minimizing long-term complications.

Even when a sexually transmitted infection causes PID, prompt diagnosis and treatment can lead to favorable outcomes. Early intervention helps to mitigate risks such as infertility, chronic pelvic pain, or progression to severe conditions like peritonitis. Therefore, recognizing and addressing PID symptoms early is essential for preserving reproductive health in adolescents.

Did You Know?

- *Painful menstruation, or dysmenorrhea, affects nearly 43–93% of adolescent girls, with severe symptoms disrupting daily activities in up to 30% of cases. Early intervention with dietary adjustments, NSAIDs, or lifestyle changes can significantly reduce discomfort.*
- *Pelvic Inflammatory Disease (PID) is rarely caused by environmental factors like sitting on cold surfaces, debunking common myths. It is most often linked to sexually transmitted infections (STIs) and requires prompt medical attention to avoid long-term complications such as infertility.*

Endometriosis

Endometriosis has become a somewhat enigmatic diagnosis, often assigned to adult women without thorough examination or justification. In developed countries, it is most frequently diagnosed among women experiencing infertility, typically between the ages of 33 and 35, when age-related fertility challenges emerge. In contrast, in regions with less advanced healthcare systems, endometriosis is sometimes overdiagnosed, as it can lead to costly laparoscopic surgeries and prolonged hormone therapies, which may not always be warranted.

The situation differs markedly when the patient is an adolescent. In teenage girls, endometriosis frequently goes undiagnosed, often dismissed as typical menstrual discomfort. Endometriosis is characterized by the presence of endometrial-like tissue outside the uterus. However, this tissue differs from the normal endometrial lining due to abnormalities in hormone receptors and its structural composition.

Endometriosis is a hormone-dependent condition primarily influenced by the maturation of egg cells. Estrogen plays a crucial role in stimulating the growth of endometriotic tissue. A key characteristic of endometriosis is its insensitivity to progesterone, a hormone that typically inhibits endometrial growth. This insensitivity results from abnormalities in the progesterone receptors within endometriotic lesions, allowing the tissue to grow unchecked.

While the exact origins of endometriosis remain unknown, numerous theories attempt to explain its development. Endometriotic lesions can affect various structures, including the ovaries, fallopian tubes, uterine ligaments, cervix, and peritoneum. Endometriosis is most diagnosed in women aged 25-29, but studies show that over half of teenage girls with severe menstrual pain (dysmenorrhea) have endometriotic lesions when evaluated laparoscopically.

Endometriosis typically develops alongside regular ovulatory cycles since endometrial growth relies on a normal hormonal balance and ovulation. This usually occurs no later than ages 17-19, emphasizing the importance of avoiding premature and aggressive interventions in younger girls.

Family history is another significant factor in adolescent endometriosis. In 35% of cases, mothers of affected girls also have a history of endometriosis, suggesting a potential genetic predisposition.

When should endometriosis be suspected in adolescents? While nearly 90% of teenage girls experience menstrual pain, the severity and pattern of pain are critical diagnostic indicators. In 62% of girls with severe dysmenorrhea, pain can be both cyclic (occurring during menstruation) and acyclic (appearing on any day of the cycle). Only 10% of girls report pain exclusively during menstruation, while 20-28% experience pain outside menstruation, with painless periods. However, more than 90% of girls with endometriosis report pain, making it the hallmark symptom of the condition.

Endometriosis can also cause gastrointestinal pain, though this is less common (34%) than dysmenorrhea, and urinary tract symptoms (2-5%) may also occur.

Adolescent endometriosis differs from the adult form of the condition. In younger patients, lesions are typically smaller (3-5 mm) and have a different morphological structure. While there is no conclusive evidence, earlier onset of endometriosis in adolescents may increase the risk of developing more severe and widespread forms of the disease later in life, often accompanied by intensified symptoms.

Understanding the unique presentation of endometriosis in adolescents is vital for timely diagnosis and management. Severe dysmenorrhea, particularly when coupled with pain outside menstruation, should prompt further investigation. With early recognition and appropriate care, the long-term impact of endometriosis on reproductive and overall health can be significantly mitigated.

Despite the presence of significant pain, diagnosing endometriosis in adolescents remains exceptionally difficult. Traditional diagnostic methods such as physical examinations, ultrasounds, and MRIs are mainly ineffective for detecting endometriosis in young girls. Healthcare providers rely on symptom documentation, dynamic observation over several menstrual cycles, and family medical history to build a clinical picture.

When all conventional dysmenorrhea treatments fail to improve the girl's condition, laparoscopic intervention may be considered. This minimally invasive procedure allows both diagnosis and treatment of endometriosis, but it is typically reserved for a small percentage of adolescents with severe forms of the disease —approximately 8%.

Currently, there are no universally accepted guidelines for diagnosing and managing endometriosis in adolescents. This diagnostic uncertainty poses significant challenges for healthcare providers and families. The complexity of endometriosis means that a girl diagnosed with the condition is likely to remain under long-term gynecological care, especially as she approaches adulthood and begins to consider pregnancy.

The absence of definitive guidelines underscores the importance of cautious, individualized care. Early recognition of symptoms and a conservative approach to intervention can help avoid unnecessary procedures while ensuring that adolescents with severe endometriosis receive the support and treatment they need.

Did You Know?

- *Endometriosis in adolescents often goes undiagnosed, as severe menstrual pain (dysmenorrhea) is frequently dismissed as "normal." Studies reveal that more than 50% of girls with severe dysmenorrhea have endometriotic lesions when evaluated laparoscopically.*
- *Unlike adult women, adolescent endometriosis lesions are typically smaller (3–5 mm) and morphologically different, but early onset can increase the risk of more severe disease later in life if left untreated.*

Cysts, Cystomas, and Other Pelvic Masses

As girls enter reproductive age and begin menstruating, they and their parents may encounter the issue of ovarian cysts, an often misunderstood phenomenon. It's important to discern to what extent ovarian masses are normal and when they might require immediate investigation and treatment.

Like other reproductive organs, the ovaries are composed of multiple tissue types, not just follicles containing eggs. Structures detected via ultrasound can have diverse histological (tissue) characteristics, making it essential to classify ovarian masses accurately.

There are two primary categories of ovarian masses: **cysts** and **cystomas.**

- **Cysts**

Cysts are retention formations — sacs filled with fluid (secretions), like small, air-filled balloons. They often arise from the follicles in functioning ovaries, which is why they are referred to as **functional cysts.** These include:

- ❖ **Follicular cysts**
- ❖ **Luteal cysts** (derived from the ovarian corpus luteum).

Functional cysts are common among adolescent girls, usually resolving spontaneously without any treatment within one to three cycles. While these cysts can grow to 8–10 cm, they pose no threat and rarely cause discomfort. Occasionally, they may rupture, releasing fluid into the pelvic cavity, which can cause brief, sharp pain due to irritation of the peritoneum.

- **Cystomas and Tissue Growths**

Cystomas, unlike cysts, involve tissue growths, "extra tissue" or "plus tissue," which can be benign or malignant. These growths are named with the suffix "*-oma*" (e.g., cystoma, lipoma, sarcoma), reflecting their nature as abnormal tissue growths. While they may accumulate fluid and occasionally exhibit hormonal activity, cystomas differ significantly from functional cysts.

There are approximately 40 types of ovarian tumors classified by cellular composition. Some of these are mistakenly labeled as cysts. Many of these tumors are malignant and require urgent evaluation and treatment. However, determining the nature of an ovarian mass is not straightforward. **Ultrasound imaging alone is insufficient for an accurate diagnosis,** as distinguishing between cysts and other types of masses often requires further diagnostic methods or histological analysis.

Adolescent girls often discover ovarian masses incidentally, as routine gynecological visits are uncommon before puberty. Sometimes, masses are only identified during surgery for unrelated conditions. Complaints such as lower abdominal pain or noticeable asymmetry in abdominal size may suggest the presence of a mass, though not necessarily of gynecological origin.

The younger the girl, the greater the likelihood that an ovarian mass may be malignant and present treatment challenges with a poorer prognosis.

Conversely, as girls grow older, most ovarian and pelvic masses are either benign or functional cysts, requiring no immediate treatment beyond observation.

Family history, particularly a record of cancer in the family, is always an important consideration when evaluating pelvic masses.

Functional cysts, such as follicular cysts, rarely require intervention. Hormonal treatment, commonly prescribed by some physicians, is generally unnecessary unless contraception is also a concern. Hormonal contraceptives, particularly high-dose options, may disrupt natural menstrual regulation processes.

Not all ovarian masses are problematic, but they do require proper evaluation. Functional cysts often resolve independently and do not need aggressive treatment, while tissue growths or tumors may necessitate closer monitoring or intervention. Accurate diagnosis is critical for determining the appropriate course of action, whether observation or treatment.

Did You Know?

- *Functional ovarian cysts, such as follicular and luteal cysts, are common in adolescent girls and typically resolve independently within 1–3 menstrual cycles, often without any treatment.*

- *Cystomas, unlike cysts, involve abnormal tissue growth and may be benign or malignant. Accurate diagnosis through imaging and histological analysis is crucial for determining their nature and necessary treatment.*

Sexually Transmitted Infections (STIs): Understanding Risks and Misconceptions

Parents often find the topic of sexually transmitted infections (STIs) confusing. Many are unaware of the various diseases that can be transmitted through different forms of sexual contact, how to diagnose these infections properly, and the available treatment options. In some countries, the diagnosis and treatment of STIs have become highly commercialized, resulting in unnecessary, repeated testing and prolonged therapies that are often misguided. However, it's important to note that most STIs today are treatable with relatively simple regimens, sometimes requiring just a single dose of medication.

A widespread but incorrect belief persists among parents that STI pathogens found in a girl's vaginal area could have been transmitted incidentally via household items such as toilet seats, potty chairs, pools, or towels. In reality, sexual transmission typically involves either direct contact (e.g., sexual intercourse) or indirect transmission from mother to child during conception or birth.

For instance, if a mother has an STI like chlamydia or gonorrhea, the infection may be transmitted to her newborn as the baby passes through the birth canal. Such cases commonly manifest as eye infections (conjunctivitis) rather than infections in the genital area. To prevent this, newborns are routinely given antibiotic eye drops immediately after birth.

Modern medicine recognizes 12 pathogens primarily transmitted through sexual contact and 23 others with partial sexual transmission potential. According to the World Health Organization (WHO), 11 out of 96 human diseases are classified as sexually transmitted. These pathogens are categorized into four main groups: viral, bacterial, fungal, and parasitic.

Viral Infections

- Hepatitis viruses (A, B, and C)
- Human Immunodeficiency Virus (HIV-1, HIV-2)

- Herpes Simplex Virus (HSV-I, HSV-II)
- Human T-lymphotropic Virus (HTLV-1)
- Human Papillomavirus (HPV)
- Cytomegalovirus (CMV)
- Epstein-Barr Virus (EBV)
- Molluscum contagiosum virus

Bacterial Infections

- *Calymmatobacterium granulomatis* (Donovanosis)
- *Chlamydia trachomatis* (types A-K and L1-L3)
- *Gardnerella vaginalis* (bacterial vaginosis)
- *Haemophilus ducreyi* (chancroid)
- *Neisseria gonorrhoeae* (gonorrhea)
- *Treponema pallidum* (syphilis)

Fungal Infections

- *Candida* species (candidiasis)
- *Histoplasma capsulatum* (histoplasmosis)

Parasitic Infections

- *Entamoeba histolytica* (amebiasis)
- *Trichomonas vaginalis* (trichomoniasis)

Ectoparasitic Infections

- *Phthirus pubis* (pubic lice)
- *Sarcoptes scabiei* (scabies)

Not all microorganisms associated with STIs directly affect the genital organs, nor do all require sexual contact for transmission. For example:

- Yeast (*Candida* species) is part of the body's normal flora and does not necessarily indicate an STI if found in the vaginal area.
- *Gardnerella vaginalis* is also a common component of normal vaginal discharge.

- Cytomegalovirus and Epstein-Barr Virus are often linked to respiratory infections and are carried by nearly 100% of adults.
- Scabies can spread through non-sexual contact, often affecting an entire household.

The presence of STI-associated microorganisms does not always indicate the presence of a sexually transmitted infection. However, there are specific scenarios where testing and evaluation are warranted:

1. **Symptoms of Pelvic Inflammatory Disease (PID):** If a child shows signs of PID, as outlined in the previous chapter, it's essential to investigate further.
2. **Suspicion or Evidence of Sexual Abuse:** Any indication of abuse necessitates a thorough medical evaluation to ensure appropriate care and intervention.

Among the various sexually transmitted infections (STIs), parents should particularly remember the following: chlamydia, gonorrhea, genital herpes, trichomoniasis, HIV, and syphilis. Human Papillomavirus (HPV) also requires attention, as it is frequently contracted with the onset of sexual activity. However, HPV has also been detected in the vaginal area of girls who have not been sexually active. It is essential to recognize that certain types of *Chlamydia* and *Neisseria* bacteria can reside in the body without causing inflammation of the reproductive organs.

STI cases peak within the young age group of 15 to 24, and adolescent girls are disproportionately affected. Statistics indicate that up to 11% of girls aged 15-19 contract STIs. This does not necessarily mean that young women are more at risk than men; instead, STIs tend to cause more discomfort and noticeable symptoms in women, leading them to seek medical attention more frequently.

Teenagers may hide their sexual activity from their parents, and if problems arise, they often turn to peers or online sources for advice rather than seeking guidance from family members. In cases of sexual abuse, a girl may feel intense fear and shame, which can prevent her from confiding in her parents. Parents must observe any changes in behavior, complaints of frequent lower abdominal pain, or recurrent urinary tract infections, as these symptoms may warrant investigation to rule out STIs.

Fostering a trusting and open environment is vital to helping adolescents feel comfortable discussing health concerns, including sensitive topics. If it becomes known that a girl has contracted an STI, reacting with anger, punishment, insults, or shameful accusations will only exacerbate her distress. Children are shaped by their upbringing, and if such an event occurs, it may reflect missed opportunities for guidance and communication. Often, the root cause lies in a lack of trust and the reluctance to address sexual education, which remains taboo in many families. Mistakes are made not only by adolescents but also by adults, who often engage in sexual relationships with multiple partners, including extramarital relationships. Unlike adults, teenagers lack the knowledge and experience necessary for STI and pregnancy prevention.

Approaching the situation with support and without judgment is essential to fostering open dialogue. This approach enables young people to make informed decisions and seek help when needed, free from fear or shame.

STI Prevention Strategies for Adolescents

Adolescents are at a higher risk for sexually transmitted infections (STIs) due to factors like biological susceptibility, limited access to healthcare, and lack of comprehensive education about sexual health. Prevention strategies tailored for this age group can significantly reduce the risk of STIs while promoting healthy behaviors and informed decision-making.

For adolescents, **abstinence**, choosing to refrain from sexual activity, is the most reliable way to prevent STIs. This includes abstaining from all forms of sexual contact, such as vaginal, oral, and anal sex. Adolescents who choose abstinence are less likely to be exposed to infectious agents during a time when they may lack access to healthcare or may not feel prepared for the responsibilities of sexual relationships. Abstinence education should focus on empowering teens with the knowledge and confidence to make this choice without judgment.

Sexually active adolescents should be educated about the consistent and correct **use of condoms**. Condoms are one of the most effective tools for preventing STIs like HIV, gonorrhea, and chlamydia. Teens often face barriers to accessing condoms due to stigma, cost, or lack of knowledge about where to obtain them. Schools, community programs, and clinics should provide free or low-cost condoms and education on their proper use. Demonstrations and discussions in a nonjudgmental setting can significantly improve adolescent knowledge and confidence in using condoms.

Both male and female condoms are effective in reducing the risk of STIs among adolescents. While male condoms are more commonly used, female condoms offer an alternative that may give young women more control over their sexual health. Educating adolescents about both options ensures they are aware of their choices and prepared for different situations.

Adolescents need to understand that while condoms are highly effective, they do not provide complete protection against all STIs. Infections like human papillomavirus (HPV) and herpes simplex virus (HSV) can spread through skin-to-skin contact, even when condoms are used. This underscores the importance of combining condom use with other preventive strategies, such as vaccination and regular testing.

Vaccination is a critical prevention tool for adolescents, as it protects them before exposure to certain infections. Pediatricians and school-based health programs ensure widespread access to these vaccines.

Parental involvement in vaccine education is essential, but teens should also be empowered to make decisions about their health with guidance from trusted healthcare providers.

For adolescents in relationships, discussing the importance of limiting sexual activity to one mutually monogamous, uninfected partner can reduce the risk of STIs. Adolescents often face pressure to engage in casual or multiple relationships, increasing their exposure to infections. Providing a safe space for teens to discuss relationships and expectations can help them make informed choices and prioritize their health.

Although needle sharing is less common among adolescents, those who engage in risky behaviors such as drug use should be educated about the dangers of sharing needles. This includes understanding the risks of HIV and hepatitis transmission through blood exposure. Adolescents should be informed about resources like needle exchange programs and harm-reduction services, which may be available in their communities.

Did You Know?

- *Adolescent girls aged 15–19 have a high risk of contracting STIs, with nearly 11% affected. Many infections remain undiagnosed due to mild or absent symptoms, emphasizing the need for early education and routine testing for sexually active teens.*
- *Condoms are one of the most effective methods for preventing STIs like HIV, gonorrhea, and chlamydia. However, infections such as HPV and herpes can still spread through skin-to-skin contact, even with condom use.*

Cervical Health, HPV Infection, and Preventing Cervical Cancer in Girls

The topic of cervical cancer prevention through HPV vaccination for girls has sparked widespread discussion and debate among parents and healthcare providers. While HPV vaccination is incorporated into public health programs in several countries and actively promoted in schools, many questions remain unanswered. Anatomically, the cervix in young girls undergoes unique physiological changes. Most young girls' cervixes exhibit what older-generation doctors often term "cervical erosion." This is ectopia or pseudo-erosion, a normal and harmless condition.

The cervix has two distinct regions: the vaginal portion and the cervical canal. The cervical canal is lined with *a glandular or columnar epithelium* that produces mucus. At the same time, the external cervix in adults is covered by *stratified squamous epithelium*, consisting of multiple cell layers. Under hormonal influences, the glandular epithelium may extend beyond the cervical canal onto the external cervix, appearing as a red, eroded area covered with clear mucus. The single-cell layer of glandular epithelium allows underlying blood vessels to show through, giving this appearance (*ectopia, ectropion*). Occasionally, mucus contains white blood cells, which may give it a white or creamy appearance, potentially mistaken as pathological discharge.

These physiological processes underscore the importance of informed decision-making regarding HPV vaccination and cervical health. Awareness of these changes can prevent unnecessary concerns and emphasize effective prevention and education.

Ectopia generally does not require treatment. In cases of intermenstrual bleeding or discomfort caused by excessive mucus discharge, surgical interventions like cauterization, laser therapy, or cryotherapy may be considered. However, these procedures are rarely performed on virgins. For sexually active adolescents, postcoital spotting may occur, necessitating the exclusion of sexually transmitted infections (STIs) before deciding on treatment. Surgical interventions carry risks, including potential cervical canal damage, which may later contribute to infertility or complications during pregnancy, such as preterm birth.

As adolescents become sexually active, they may encounter another issue —HPV infection. Remarkably, 99% of girls are unaware if they have contracted HPV, and most women will never know.

Over 130 types of HPV are known to inhabit human skin and mucous membranes, though no single individual hosts all types. Some HPV strains are transient, while others may persist lifelong. Most HPV infections are harmless, causing minimal to no issues for the host. However, more than 40 HPV types can infect the anogenital tract, raising public health concerns.

HPV is associated with cervical cancer, though its role in causing the disease remains unclear. HPV types are categorized as "high-risk" (oncogenic) or "low-risk" (non-oncogenic). High-risk types include 16, 18, 31, 33, 35, 39, 45, 51, 52, 56, 58, 59, 68, and 82, with types 16 and 18 accounting for 70% of precancerous and cancerous cases. Low-risk types, such as 6 and 11, are linked to 90% of genital warts.

Understanding HPV's classifications allows parents and girls to approach HPV-related health issues with less fear and more excellent knowledge, especially when considering vaccination and preventive measures.

By the age of 30, over 70% of men and women have been infected with HPV at least once, and 45–50% of women aged 20–24 have an active HPV infection, primarily among students in vocational schools and universities. Among urban teenage girls, 64% have HPV DNA detected in vaginal secretions within two years of beginning sexual activity, with nearly one-third infected after their first sexual encounter. HPV infection rates significantly decrease after age 30.

Even among 20% of young girls who have never engaged in vaginal intercourse, HPV is found in vaginal secretions and on the vulva, indicating that the virus can inhabit these areas without sexual activity.

Despite these statistics, there is cause for optimism. In 90% of infected women, HPV clears entirely within two years, often within 3 to 6 months. The presence of HPV in vaginal secretions does not necessitate treatment, as no specific therapy exists for HPV. Additionally, 99% of women exposed to oncogenic HPV types will never develop cervical cancer.

Cervical cancer remains a rare disease, and its incidence is even lower among girls and adolescents. Its development is usually unrelated to HPV infection in this age group. Consequently, detecting HPV in a child's vaginal secretions should not incite panic or lead to unnecessary interventions.

Among adolescents and young women who have started sexual activity, genital warts caused by non-oncogenic HPV types are commonly observed. These warts can cause itching, discomfort, and dissatisfaction with the appearance of the external genitalia. They often appear in areas of friction from tight underwear or clothing and may bleed due to constant irritation. Warts can be removed through chemical or surgical methods, but a qualified doctor should always perform this. Self-treatment can lead to burns or scarring of the vulva and perineum, exacerbating the issue.

HPV testing is not typically recommended for girls or adolescents under 25 years of age. Here's why:

1. **HPV infections are common and transient in younger individuals:**

Most HPV infections in adolescents and young women are temporary and are cleared by the immune system within 1–2 years. Testing during this period may detect transient infections unlikely to cause long-term harm or cervical changes.

2. **Cervical cancer risk is extremely low in this age group:**

Cervical cancer is rare in adolescents and young women under 25, and cervical screening programs focus on detecting precancerous changes rather than transient HPV infections.

3. **Potential for overtreatment:**

Detecting HPV in younger individuals could lead to unnecessary follow-ups, anxiety, and interventions for conditions that might resolve without treatment.

HPV testing is usually integrated into cervical cancer screening programs, often starting at age 25 or 30, depending on the guidelines of the specific country. In some countries, HPV testing is combined with a Pap smear (cytology) for women aged 30 and older, as persistent HPV infections are more likely to indicate a risk for cervical precancer and cancer. Suppose a young girl (e.g., under 25) has specific risk factors, such as a history of sexual abuse, multiple sexual partners, or other high-risk behaviors. In that case, her healthcare provider might consider testing or closer monitoring on a case-by-case basis.

HPV testing may be conducted if a Pap smear reveals abnormal cervical cells (e.g., atypical squamous cells of undetermined significance, ASC-US), regardless of age.

Now, turning to HPV vaccination for the prevention of cervical cancer, the topic is surrounded by myths and misunderstandings. One prevalent myth is that this "cancer vaccine" causes menstrual cycle disruptions and future infertility. These claims are entirely false. First, this is not a vaccine against cancer itself but rather against HPV infection. Second, it is entirely safe for a girl's reproductive health and future as a woman, although, like all vaccines, it may have some side effects.

Currently, there are three types of prophylactic HPV vaccines available:

1. **Bivalent vaccine**: Protects against HPV types 16 and 18.
2. **Quadrivalent vaccine**: This vaccine provides protection against HPV types 6, 11, 16, and 18. It does not contain antibiotics or preservatives.
3. **Nine-valent vaccine**: This vaccine targets nine HPV types: 6, 11, 16, 18, 31, 33, 45, 52, and 58. Like the quadrivalent vaccine, it is free from antibiotics and preservatives.

All three vaccines are administered in a three-dose schedule and approved for females and males aged 9 to 45. However, debates persist about the vaccine's duration of effectiveness, the ideal age for administration, its high cost, and potential side effects.

Studies indicate that the vaccine provides protective effects for 6–8 years when used correctly. If children are vaccinated at the recommended age of 9, this protection may expire by age 19. This raises questions about the timing of vaccination, particularly for girls who may not begin sexual activity until later. Anonymous surveys and studies suggest that modern girls in developed countries tend to delay their first sexual contact to an average age of 18.5–19.5 years. This delay is attributed mainly to improved sexual education, better access to accurate information about the consequences of early sexual activity, and awareness of contraception and STI prevention.

The onset of sexual activity also depends on socioeconomic conditions. Girls from lower socioeconomic backgrounds are at higher risk for STIs, including HPV, teenage pregnancies, and sexual violence. This demographic is the most in need of vaccination at puberty. Yet, these adolescents often remain unvaccinated due to the vaccine's high cost and the lack of inclusion in government-funded health programs.

Some doctors advocate for a two-dose vaccination schedule, which reduces costs, but even this remains unaffordable for many families. Additionally, there are no clear recommendations about revaccination after 10 years, such as which vaccine to use, the appropriate dose, or how often to administer it.

Further research and reliable data are necessary to address the many unanswered questions about HPV, its prevention, and its role in cervical cancer prevention. For instance, it is well-documented that hormonal contraceptive use and smoking increase the risk of developing cervical cancer. Yet, this information is rarely communicated to teenage girls and young women. Education on preventing dangerous diseases should begin in schools and encompass more than just vaccination.

Many healthcare professionals, scientists, and educators agree that improving sexual education in schools is critical. Comprehensive education could lower rates of STIs, teenage pregnancies, and sexual violence, and it would also mitigate many other negative consequences of early sexual activity that can surface later in adulthood.

The decision to vaccinate a child against HPV should be a conscious and informed one made by parents and adolescents together. Unfortunately, in some cases, fear tactics have been used to coerce vaccination, targeting parents and children alike. Such practices are unethical and, in some instances, may be legally punishable.

Vaccination has undeniably saved millions of lives by preventing life-threatening diseases such as polio, measles, and smallpox, profoundly transforming global public health. However, the case for HPV vaccination, which targets an infection that is not inherently fatal for the vast majority of those infected, requires a more nuanced approach. While HPV is linked to cervical cancer and other anogenital cancers, these conditions develop in only a tiny percentage of those infected and often over decades, giving ample time for monitoring and intervention. Thus, the justification for widespread HPV vaccination hinges on its potential to reduce the burden of HPV-related diseases, including precancerous lesions and genital warts, which can affect the quality of life and require medical treatment.

To maximize the benefits of HPV vaccination, it is critical to establish clear, evidence-based guidelines that consider the vaccine's cost, accessibility, and long-term effectiveness. This includes identifying the most appropriate age groups for vaccination, determining the necessity and timing of booster doses, and understanding the vaccine's impact on HPV transmission and herd immunity.

Furthermore, ensuring equitable access to the vaccine, especially in low-income and underserved populations where the burden of HPV-related diseases is often highest, is essential for achieving public health goals. Transparent communication about the vaccine's benefits, limitations, and potential side effects is equally important to build public trust and encourage informed decision-making. By addressing these factors, HPV vaccination can become a more effective and widely accepted tool in the broader strategy for cancer prevention.

Did You Know?

- *Over 70% of men and women will contract HPV by age 30, with many infections clearing on their own within 2 years, thanks to the immune system.*
- *Cervical cancer is rare in adolescents and young women, and the presence of HPV in vaginal secretions in this age group usually does not require treatment.*

Contraception and Adolescents

With the onset of puberty, adolescents often begin to explore intimacy, a process that usually starts with a desire for affection through hugs and kisses. As they grow older, this curiosity frequently progresses to physical relationships. However, boys and girls typically approach sexual activity with different motivations and expectations. For many boys, engaging in sexual activity serves as a form of self-affirmation, a way to assert their maturity and transition into manhood. For girls, sexual involvement is often an emotional response, a desire to please someone they care deeply about. Many fear that rejecting a partner's advances might jeopardize their relationship.

Unfortunately, most adolescents lack the comprehensive knowledge needed to make informed decisions about sexual health. Many are unaware of how conception occurs, the risks of sexually transmitted infections (STIs), or how to use contraception effectively. Even when some information is available, adolescents often act invincibly, believing, "This won't happen to me!" This belief, combined with a tendency toward maximalism and rigid thinking, frequently leads to poor decision-making and a disregard for potential consequences.

Sexual education remains a taboo subject in many families. Parents often feel uncomfortable addressing intimate topics and may lack the knowledge or resources to provide accurate information. In addition, cultural, religious, and societal restrictions can discourage discussions about sexual relationships. Regardless of these barriers, children and adolescents must understand that sex is not just a natural part of life but also a significant responsibility with profound implications for their health and future.

Research shows that contraception usage among adolescents under 18–19 years old remains alarmingly low. Despite widespread awareness of various contraceptive methods, many teens fail to use them consistently. The two most common reasons for unprotected sexual activity are alcohol consumption, leading to impaired judgment—and pressure from a partner. Many girls enter sexual relationships without preparation, lacking both the moral confidence and practical knowledge needed to assert control over their choices. This unpreparedness often leads to unplanned pregnancies and increased vulnerability to STIs.

Studies reveal that irregular sexual activity also contributes to inconsistent contraceptive use. Adolescents often engage in spontaneous encounters where condoms or other contraceptives are unavailable. Even when a girl carries a condom, it may go unused due to the reluctance to "interrupt the moment."

In some countries, schools have introduced anonymous counseling centers to provide adolescents with information about sexual relationships, distribute free condoms, and offer emergency contraception when necessary. These initiatives have successfully reduced teenage pregnancy rates, lowered abortion rates, and curbed STI infections. However, the availability of such resources remains inconsistent worldwide, leaving many adolescents without the guidance they need.

Children often ask their parents, "How was I born?" from an early age. Parents respond in various ways, ranging from fanciful tales about storks and cabbage patches to straightforward explanations about reproduction. Unfortunately, many adolescents begin their sexual lives before acquiring even basic knowledge about contraception or STI prevention. Inadequate sexual education in schools exacerbates this problem, leaving young people vulnerable.

Parents, too, often lack comprehensive knowledge about contraception. Consequently, the responsibility for educating adolescents frequently falls to healthcare professionals. Adolescents should have access to age-appropriate, accurate, and judgment-free guidance on contraception provided by both educators and healthcare providers.

Contraceptive Methods

Contraceptive methods can be categorized based on their mechanisms of action:

- Preventing egg maturation: Hormonal methods.
- Blocking sperm-egg contact: Barrier methods.
- Permanently halting reproductive function: Sterilization.
- Preventing fertilized egg implantation: Hormonal methods or intrauterine devices (IUDs).

- ***Calendar Method***

The calendar method involves tracking menstrual cycles to predict fertile days and avoid intercourse during these times. This method is highly unreliable for adolescents due to the irregularity of their cycles. However, teaching young girls to observe their body's hormonal changes can help them better understand their reproductive health.

- ***Withdrawal (Coitus Interruptus)***

This method requires the male partner to withdraw before ejaculation. It is one of the least reliable methods, especially for inexperienced adolescents, as it requires significant control and timing. Withdrawal does not protect against STIs and is generally not recommended.

- ***Barrier Methods***

Barrier methods include male and female condoms, cervical caps, diaphragms, and spermicidal sponges. Male condoms are affordable, effective, and protect against many STIs, making them a highly recommended option for adolescents. Even if a girl uses another contraceptive method, she should always carry condoms for backup protection. Spermicides alone are less reliable and do not protect against STIs.

- ***Hormonal Methods***

Hormonal contraceptives suppress ovulation and alter the cervical mucus and endometrial lining to prevent pregnancy. Options include pills, patches, vaginal rings, implants, injections, and hormonal IUDs. While these methods are effective, they require consistent use, something many adolescents struggle with. Cost can also be prohibitive for young people without financial independence.

- ***Intrauterine Devices (IUDs)***

IUDs, both hormonal and non-hormonal, are effective and safe for adolescents and women who have not given birth. They are cost-effective and provide long-term protection against pregnancy. However, IUD insertion requires a healthcare professional and should be discussed thoroughly with the adolescent and her parents.

- ***Emergency Contraception***

Emergency contraception is designed for use after unprotected intercourse. High-dose progestins, such as levonorgestrel, are effective within 72 hours, while IUDs can be inserted up to seven days after intercourse. Emergency contraception should not replace regular contraceptive methods, as frequent use can disrupt menstrual cycles. Adolescents should be educated about its availability and proper use.

- ***Abstinence and Alternative Practices***

While abstinence is the only foolproof method for preventing pregnancy and STIs, it is not a realistic choice for all adolescents. Many young people turn to anal or oral sex as alternatives to vaginal intercourse, believing these practices will preserve their virginity or prevent pregnancy. However, these practices still carry significant risks for STI transmission. Condom use is essential in these situations.

One lesser-known consequence of hormonal contraceptive use is the **syndrome of hyper-suppression of pituitary gonadotropic function**. This condition involves significantly suppressing gonadotropin production, disrupting the hypothalamic-pituitary-ovarian axis. Adolescents are particularly vulnerable to this syndrome because their reproductive systems are still maturing. After discontinuing hormonal contraceptives, it may take several months or even longer for menstrual cycles to normalize, often leading to a cycle of repeated prescriptions and dependency.

Parents and adolescents must understand that no contraceptive method is perfect or free from side effects. Adolescents should receive comprehensive education on the risks and benefits of each process to make informed choices. Prolonged or irregular use of hormonal medications can interfere with the development of the hypothalamic-pituitary-ovarian axis, affecting menstrual regularity.

Creating a supportive environment for open discussions about sexual health can empower adolescents to make responsible decisions. Schools, healthcare providers, and parents must collaborate to provide young people with the tools they need to navigate the complexities of intimacy and contraception responsibly.

Did You Know?

- *Adolescents are often unaware that inconsistent contraceptive use and unprotected sexual activity are the leading causes of unplanned pregnancies and STIs, with many cases resulting from a lack of preparation or impaired judgment during spontaneous encounters.*
- *Barrier methods like condoms not only prevent pregnancy but also protect against most STIs, making them one of the most effective and accessible options for adolescents.*

Teenage Pregnancy

Adolescent pregnancy, though less common in modern societies than in the past, remains a critical issue with profound physical, emotional, and social implications. Historically, girls as young as 14–16 were often married; in some regions, even younger marriages were the norm. By age 20, many women had already given birth to multiple children. However, the high rates of pregnancy complications and maternal mortality among such young mothers were rarely addressed in societies dominated by cultural and religious traditions. Even today, in some parts of the world, child marriages are still considered acceptable and are legally permitted, perpetuating this cycle.

In contrast, in many countries today, the average age of marriage and planned pregnancies has risen to around 30 years. Despite this, unplanned pregnancies among adolescents remain prevalent, particularly in communities with low socioeconomic status. These pregnancies are often a result of limited access to contraception, poor education, and higher rates of sexual violence or coercion.

The actual rate of adolescent pregnancies is challenging to determine, as many families handle these situations discreetly, sometimes resorting to unsafe, illegal abortions. In the United States, approximately 27 out of every 1,000 births occur in mothers aged 15–19. However, the introduction of sex education programs and anonymous counseling centers has significantly reduced unplanned pregnancies and abortions among teenagers over the past 25 years.

Historically, the peak of teenage pregnancies occurred after World War II, but rates have since declined considerably. Nonetheless, about 17% of adolescents still experience repeat unplanned pregnancies. In Europe, adolescent pregnancy rates are notably lower than in the United States and other regions.

For many adolescents, discovering they are pregnant is a shock, often occurring too late for them to consider terminating the pregnancy. Many girls are unaware of the early signs of pregnancy.

Irregular menstrual cycles, which are common in adolescence, may cause a missed period to go unnoticed. Symptoms such as nausea and vomiting, typical of pregnancy, do not affect all women and may be attributed to other factors like poor nutrition. Weakness, mood swings, and breast sensitivity are common in adolescents for various reasons and may not raise concern.

If a missed period occurs, mainly if a girl previously had regular cycles, pregnancy should be ruled out. Home pregnancy tests, available at most pharmacies, are highly sensitive and reliable after a delay of at least seven days.

Risks of Adolescent Pregnancy

Pregnancy during adolescence places significant physical and emotional strain on a body that is still developing. Young mothers often face financial instability, a lack of partner or parental support, and the challenge of balancing education with their new responsibilities. Many are forced to drop out of school, and some face verbal or physical abuse from family members who view the pregnancy as a source of shame.

Physically, adolescent pregnancies are associated with higher risks of complications, including high blood pressure, preeclampsia, preterm birth, and low birth weight. Babies born to teenage mothers are more likely to experience intrauterine growth restriction and weigh between 1,500–2,500 grams at birth.

Adolescent mothers are also at a higher risk of contracting sexually transmitted infections (STIs), which can severely impact both the mother and the baby during delivery. Additionally, teenage mothers are more likely to engage in behaviors like smoking, alcohol consumption, and drug use, all of which can harm fetal development and maternal health.

Postpartum depression is more common in teenage mothers, driven by feelings of isolation, shame, and despair. Many young mothers face neglect or abandonment by friends and family, exacerbating their sense of social isolation.

Supporting an Adolescent Mother

If your daughter becomes pregnant during adolescence, it is essential to approach the situation with empathy and support. Scolding, blaming, or isolating her will only add to her stress and emotional burden. Instead, offer emotional, financial, and practical assistance to help her navigate the challenges ahead.

A confirmed pregnancy diagnosis should be followed by regular medical care to monitor the health of both the mother and the baby. Psychological support, whether from a psychotherapist, psychologist, or social worker, can help the young mother cope with the changes and responsibilities of pregnancy and motherhood.

It is also crucial to discuss the girl's educational and career plans to ensure she can continue her education and build a future for herself and her child. Daycare or preschool options should be explored to facilitate her return to school. Forced marriage, often suggested to "hide the shame," is not recommended, as such unions frequently end in separation, causing prolonged suffering for all involved.

No matter the circumstances, it is essential to remember that your daughter is still your child — a reflection of your care and upbringing. She will need your guidance and support more than ever. Together, you can navigate the challenges of adolescent pregnancy and help her build a stable and fulfilling future.

Did You Know?

- *Adolescent pregnancies are more common in regions with limited access to contraception and poor sexual education, highlighting the importance of awareness programs and counseling.*
- *Teenage mothers face higher risks of complications such as preterm birth, low birth weight, and postpartum depression, making regular medical care and emotional support essential.*

Breasts and Related Issues

Breast development and related issues during adolescence often bring about concerns for both girls and their parents. While most conditions are benign and part of normal development, some may require medical attention. Here is an overview of the most common breast-related issues in adolescents:

- ***Breast Size***

Asymmetric breast growth is common during puberty. It is normal for one breast to grow faster than the other, with most asymmetry evening out by the end of puberty. However, it is common for one breast, often the right, to remain slightly larger due to natural bodily asymmetry.

If the size difference is significant or persists, medical evaluation may be necessary to rule out conditions such as cysts or fibroadenomas.

For thin girls with limited fatty tissue, breasts may remain small until later in puberty or even during pregnancy. If menstrual cycles are regular despite small breast size, there is typically no cause for concern.

In recent years, there has been an increase in breast reduction surgeries among adolescents. Such procedures are not recommended until after a woman has completed childbirth and breastfeeding, except in cases where large breasts cause physical discomfort, such as neck or back pain, or interfere with daily activities.

- ***Nipple Discharge***

Adolescents should not generally experience nipple discharge, but when it occurs, it is not always a sign of a medical problem. Clear or milky discharge is often linked to elevated prolactin levels, which can result from stress, sleep deprivation, smoking, or thyroid conditions.

Discharge of other colors, such as green, bloody, purulent, or yellow, requires a medical evaluation to rule out underlying conditions, though serious illnesses are rare.

- ***Breast Pain***

Breast pain during adolescence is commonly linked to hormonal fluctuations throughout the menstrual cycle. In the first half of the cycle, breast cells grow in response to estrogen. In the second phase, rising progesterone levels can lead to swelling and tenderness. If pregnancy does not occur, these cells undergo programmed cell death (apoptosis), which can cause mild inflammation and discomfort.

This cyclic breast pain, often associated with premenstrual syndrome (PMS), is a normal physiological phenomenon. Explaining these changes to adolescents can alleviate anxiety about the pain.

Properly fitting bras are essential to minimize discomfort, especially during the second half of the cycle. Girls should avoid wearing bras to bed and opt for loose, comfortable sleepwear.

- ***Breast Lumps***

Lumps in the breasts are common during adolescence and are typically benign. Fibroadenomas are the most frequent findings during breast examinations or ultrasounds. These benign growths are not harmful, though they can cause discomfort. They may appear in one or both breasts and often require only observation unless they cause significant symptoms, in which case surgical removal may be considered.

Cystic-fibrous changes, often mischaracterized as "mastopathy," are another common finding. These changes can cause localized firmness, swelling, and pain but do not lead to cancer.

- ***Infections and Inflammation***

Mastitis, an infection of the breast tissue, is rare in non-lactating adolescents. However, physical trauma such as cuts, piercings, or injuries can introduce bacteria into the breast, leading to inflammation. Symptoms include redness, swelling, pain, and fever. Antibiotics are typically effective in treating these infections.

While most breast-related issues in adolescence are benign and resolve naturally, a healthcare provider should evaluate any persistent or concerning symptoms. Open communication and education about breast development can help alleviate anxiety and promote proactive health management.

Did You Know?

- *Breast asymmetry during adolescence is entirely normal and often resolves by the end of puberty, though slight differences may persist into adulthood.*
- *Cyclic breast pain, often linked to hormonal changes, is a standard part of adolescence and usually decreases over time as hormonal cycles stabilize.*

Nutrition for Girls

Proper nutrition is a concern for parents from the earliest days of a child's life, beginning with questions about breastfeeding, formula, and transitioning to solid foods. As children grow, especially girls entering adolescence, questions about specific dietary needs and the impact of nutrition on development arise. Although there are no significant differences in dietary requirements between healthy girls and boys, puberty introduces unique hormonal changes in girls that can influence their nutritional needs and gastrointestinal function.

With the onset of menstrual cycles, hormonal fluctuations affect various bodily functions, including digestion. During the first half of the cycle, increased motility speeds up digestion, while reduced motility can lead to constipation in the second half. To address this, girls should consume more fiber-rich foods, such as fruits, vegetables, and whole grains, and drink adequate water, particularly in the second phase of the cycle. Reducing sugary drinks and processed foods can also help.

No specific foods are restricted for healthy girls, apart from alcohol-containing products.

Observations across diverse cultures show that dietary diversity does not hinder growth or development as long as essential nutrients are provided.

Adolescence often marks the beginning of serious nutritional challenges. Girls are frequently influenced by societal ideals of beauty, usually modeled after celebrities and fashion trends. Over the past five decades, these ideals have shifted toward thinner body types, leading to widespread body image concerns and, in some cases, eating disorders.

- About 90% of all eating disorders occur in women.
- Approximately 80% of teenage girls fear gaining weight.
- One in seven women will experience an eating disorder in their lifetime.

- Among adolescents, 40%, and by some estimates, one in three girls, believe they are overweight, with 60% actively trying to lose weight.

Unlike boys, who tend to address weight concerns through impulsive exercise routines, girls often resort to fasting, extreme dieting, or other potentially harmful methods.

One alarming trend is the "alcohol diet," where adolescents consume alcohol instead of food, believing it provides sufficient calories while avoiding weight gain. This practice is not only dangerous but can quickly lead to alcohol dependency, malnutrition, and severe health consequences.

Adolescents must understand that the body requires a balanced intake of nutrients, including carbohydrates, fats, and proteins, to function properly and maintain healthy cell and tissue structures.

Girls often emulate the behaviors of older women in their lives, such as mothers or sisters. In developed countries, over 45% of women aged 30–35 are on diets, contributing to the normalization of restrictive eating habits. In the U.S. alone, the diet industry generates $40 billion annually, yet it often fails to address the root causes of obesity.

What Girls Should Know About Weight

1. **Weight-to-Height Ratio**: Maintaining a balanced weight-to-height ratio is essential for overall health.
2. **Growth and Weight Management**: Genetics largely determine height, while weight can be managed through diet and activity within healthy limits.
3. **Body Fat Percentage**: A healthy body fat percentage (17–24%) supports reproductive and general health. Both excessive and insufficient fat can disrupt bodily functions.
4. **Nutritional and Emotional Stress**: Malnutrition and stress, particularly from drastic weight changes, can lead to menstrual irregularities and infertility.

Eating Disorders

Eating disorders are mental health conditions that disrupt normal eating behaviors and metabolism. These disorders often arise from negative body image and can result in inadequate or excessive weight relative to height. Common eating disorders include:

- **Anorexia nervosa**: Extreme food restriction and fear of weight gain.
- **Bulimia nervosa**: Binge eating followed by purging through vomiting or excessive exercise.
- **Pica**: Eating non-food substances.
- **Rumination disorder**: Repeated regurgitation and re-chewing of food.
- **Binge eating disorder**: Consuming large quantities of food in a short period, often accompanied by guilt.

Parents may observe disordered eating behaviors, such as excessive dieting, refusal to eat, rapid weight fluctuations, or compulsive overeating. While such behaviors often stem from psychological factors, they are sometimes misdiagnosed and treated by pediatricians or gastroenterologists before their underlying mental health roots are addressed.

Proper support, including education about healthy eating habits and open communication, is critical to addressing these issues and preventing long-term complications.

- **Pica**

Pica, the consumption of non-food substances, is a condition often observed in early childhood. Young children naturally explore their environment by putting objects into their mouths, sometimes developing a preference for non-edible items such as glue, dirt, toothpaste, paint, pet food, perfume, feces, paper, stones, or garbage.

Pica is most common in children aged 1 to 6 years and may either be a transient phase of curiosity or a persistent behavior linked to underlying factors like malnutrition, intellectual disabilities, or poor maternal relationships.

Determining whether pica is a normal developmental phase or a more serious issue requires careful observation over at least one month. Frequent or prolonged consumption of non-food items can lead to significant health risks, including poisoning, foodborne infections, or digestive blockages. Intervention from a child psychiatrist or medical professional is essential in such cases.

- **Rumination Disorder**

Rumination disorder is characterized by the repeated regurgitation of partially digested food, which is re-chewed, swallowed, or spit out. Unlike vomiting, this behavior is deliberate and may occur multiple times daily.

The exact cause of rumination is unclear, though it is often linked to stress or poor mother-child relationships. It may also result from congenital gastrointestinal abnormalities, such as lower esophageal or stomach enlargement, pylorospasm, esophageal atresia, or achalasia. Behavioral factors like thumb-sucking or nail-biting can also contribute to its development.

Persistent rumination can cause bad breath, cracked lips, weight loss, and digestive disorders. In severe cases, food particles may enter the bronchial system, leading to respiratory infections. Medical evaluation is essential to identify potential gastrointestinal or psychological causes when rumination is observed. Depending on the underlying condition, treatment may include medications, surgery, or psychotherapy.

- **Psychogenic Overeating**

Occasional overeating during times of stress is common, but psychogenic overeating refers to a chronic and impulsive pattern of consuming large amounts of food due to emotional or psychological triggers. This behavior is often characterized by:

- Rapid consumption of large quantities of food in short
- periods.
- Eating without hunger.

- Developing a dependence on overeating for comfort.
- Late-night eating, sometimes without memory of the food consumed.

Psychogenic overeating is often accompanied by feelings of guilt, shame, or disgust, creating a cycle of conflict where the individual does not want to eat but feels powerless to stop. Unlike bulimia, this condition does not involve purging.

Psychogenic overeating is most seen in women and adolescents and is often accompanied by symptoms like insomnia, depression, and fatigue. While the exact cause remains unclear, it is frequently linked to social, cultural, and psychological factors, and in rare cases, it may involve dysfunction in the hypothalamus.

Parents play a significant role in shaping eating behaviors, often inadvertently associating food with comfort or rewards through phrases like:

"Are you upset? Have a cookie!"

"Hurt your leg? Here's some candy."

"Finish your homework, and you'll get ice cream."

Such behaviors can establish unhealthy emotional relationships with food. Adolescents, particularly girls, often experience heightened emotional responses and anxieties about self-image, which may exacerbate tendencies toward overeating.

Psychogenic overeating can lead to weight gain, obesity, and associated physical and mental health challenges. Addressing the root causes through psychological support and promoting healthy coping mechanisms is crucial.

Treatment for psychogenic overeating requires a comprehensive approach involving a psychotherapist, dietitian, pediatrician, and the active involvement of parents. If depression is present, antidepressants may be prescribed, and in some cases, appetite-suppressing medications are used.

The cornerstone of treatment is psychotherapy, which focuses on identifying stressors and teaching the child healthier ways to cope with negative emotions and life events without resorting to overeating. This gradual process demands patience and commitment from everyone involved, especially the child and their family.

- **Bulimia**

Bulimia is a severe eating disorder characterized by cycles of undereating, overeating, and self-induced vomiting. This behavior often stems from a distorted perception of one's body and an intense fear of weight gain.

Several signs may indicate bulimia in adolescents, including frequent overeating episodes, repeated trips to the bathroom immediately after meals, the smell of vomit, and the use of laxatives or diuretics. Girls with bulimia may also engage in excessive physical exercise, often to the point of exhaustion. Other symptoms include social withdrawal, secretive behaviors, and a noticeable reduction in dietary variety.

Bulimia affects approximately 1–2% of adolescent girls and young women, primarily between the ages of 13 and 20. It is overwhelmingly more common in females, with 80% of cases occurring in women. Depression accompanies about 70% of bulimia cases, and 10–20% of individuals struggle with the disorder for more than a decade.

Frequent vomiting poses significant health risks. It disrupts the body's water and electrolyte balance, which can impair cardiovascular function due to dehydration and the loss of essential electrolytes like sodium and potassium. In severe cases, this imbalance can be fatal.

Diagnosing bulimia is particularly challenging, as extreme weight loss is not always present. Weight may be lower than average but not critically so, which can mask the condition.

The primary treatment for bulimia is psychotherapy, which helps the individual address underlying emotional and psychological factors contributing to the disorder. Antidepressants are often used in conjunction with therapy to manage symptoms of depression and improve overall mental health.

Bulimia is a deeply ingrained and dangerous condition, and most individuals require professional help and long-term support to overcome it.

- **Anorexia**

Anorexia is one of the most severe and life-threatening eating disorders, marked by the highest mortality rate among mental health conditions, including deaths by suicide. Recovery is observed in only about half of those who develop the disorder.

Anorexia is characterized by extremely low body weight, an intense fear of gaining weight, and an obsessive desire to be thin, leading to severe restriction of food intake.

Body mass index (BMI) is commonly used in adults to assess whether an individual's weight falls within a healthy range. BMI is calculated as:

$$\textbf{BMI} = \textbf{Weight (kg)} / [\textbf{Height (m)}]^2$$

Anorexia is generally diagnosed when a BMI falls below 16. Growth patterns and weight gain in children and adolescents differ significantly from those of adults, so BMI is not a reliable measure for evaluating their health. Instead, pediatricians use growth charts that compare a child's measurements to standardized percentiles. Weight below the 5th percentile is considered critically low and indicative of potential health risks.

Treating anorexia is exceptionally challenging, as no specific medications exist to cure the condition directly. Medical professionals often focus on addressing the physical consequences of anorexia, such as severe electrolyte imbalances, metabolic disruptions, and cardiovascular complications, all of which can pose immediate threats to life.

Anorexia is deeply rooted in mental health issues stemming from a distorted perception of one's body. As a result, psychiatrists and psychotherapists are essential in the treatment process. Adolescents and women with anorexia often require hospitalization to stabilize their physical and mental health.

Psychotherapy plays a central role in treatment and may involve various approaches, including individual therapy, group therapy, and family therapy. Family involvement is crucial, as recovery is nearly impossible without consistent support and encouragement from parents and close relatives.

Parents should monitor their child's eating habits and attitudes toward food and weight, mainly if there are noticeable signs of excessive weight loss or preoccupation with body image. Engaging in open and empathetic discussions about societal beauty standards and the importance of a healthy relationship with food can help prevent the onset of anorexia or detect its progression early.

Anorexia is a complex and persistent disorder requiring a multidisciplinary approach to treatment. Early intervention and ongoing support significantly improve the chances of recovery.

Did You Know?

- *Over 80% of teenage girls fear gaining weight, with many attempting extreme dieting methods, which can lead to serious physical and mental health consequences.*
- *Eating disorders such as anorexia and bulimia often stem from societal pressure and distorted body image, but they can be effectively managed with early intervention and professional support.*

Appearance, Makeup, and Plastic Surgery

Women are inherently drawn to mirrors, often spending considerable time examining their reflections, and girls are no exception. As puberty begins, girls naturally pay more attention to their appearance, motivated by a desire to look attractive, particularly to the opposite sex.

Interestingly, this desire is rooted in reproductive instincts and hormonal changes. During ovulation, hormonal fluctuations influence women to wear brighter clothing, apply makeup, and accentuate features they find attractive. Even adolescent girls, once they begin menstruating, exhibit mood and behavioral variations depending on their menstrual cycle phase, subtly reflecting these instinctual patterns.

Girls often seek inspiration from their mothers, idols, or popular peers. The individuality that shapes personal style—choices in clothing, hairstyles, and accessories—typically develops after puberty as girls gain confidence in expressing their unique preferences.

Adolescents often become preoccupied with their appearance, worrying about acne, body hair on their legs, arms, or face, asymmetrical breast sizes, and other perceived imperfections. These concerns are not purely superficial but are intertwined with developing self-esteem and the social pressures of adolescence.

Interest in cosmetics and perfume emerges early, often sparked by watching mothers or older siblings. Young girls may ask their mothers to paint their fingernails or toenails, intrigued by manicures and pedicures. Many experiment secretly with their mothers' makeup, perfumes, earrings, necklaces, and shoes, exploring the transformative power of adornment.

As they age, girls' preferences shift toward what is popular among their peers, viewing their mothers' styles as outdated or "uncool." This divergence is a response to trends and part of asserting independence. While some mothers adapt to modern trends, many adolescents focus on separating themselves from adults, striving to discover their identity.

There is no universal answer to when girls should start using makeup. Today, cosmetics are marketed to younger audiences, and makeup use has become common for activities such as dance performances, sports competitions, beauty pageants, and school plays. However, the regular use of makeup often begins during adolescence.

Teenagers frequently use makeup and hairstyles as forms of self-expression. For some, bold makeup and unconventional hair colors signal an effort to express individuality, particularly if they feel restricted at home or overlooked by loved ones. Such styles can also be a way to align with trends or gain attention from their peers. It's worth noting that the makeup teenagers use is often of low quality due to their limited financial resources. This impacts the longevity and appearance of their makeup and can also pose risks to their skin health, especially with frequent use.

If your child decides to start using makeup, it's wise to guide them in selecting high-quality, hypoallergenic products. While "natural" cosmetics do not exist, many products now include natural ingredients, offering safer options for young skin.

Few resources exist specifically for teenagers who correctly use cosmetics and perfumes, yet teaching them proper techniques is vital. Adolescents often rely on peer influence, prioritizing trends over comfort or health. This can lead to excessive or inappropriate use of makeup, potentially causing skin irritation, clogged pores, or an overly artificial appearance.

Parents and guardians play a crucial role in guiding teens through their exploration of cosmetics. Helping girls understand the importance of proper skincare, moderation, and choosing age-appropriate styles fosters healthy habits and protects their developing skin.

Additionally, parents can use this opportunity to have open, judgment-free discussions about self-esteem and the influence of societal beauty standards. Highlighting that makeup should enhance rather than define their natural beauty can instill confidence and encourage self-expression without succumbing to external pressures.

By offering support and guidance, parents can help girls navigate the complexities of adolescence while allowing them the freedom to explore their evolving identity through makeup and style.

Teenagers and Plastic Surgery

Adolescence is a time of heightened self-awareness and insecurity, during which many teenagers become overly critical of their appearance. They may fixate on perceived defects and desire to "fix" them, believing that doing so will enhance their self-esteem or social standing. The allure of plastic surgery, often glamorized by celebrities and social media, has become particularly strong for some teenagers.

Plastic and cosmetic surgery, however, is expensive and carries inherent risks and long-term consequences. Despite these factors, many teenagers seek surgical solutions to their perceived flaws. In the United States alone, nearly 300,000 girls under the age of 19 undergo plastic surgery annually.

The types of plastic surgery commonly sought by teenagers include:

- **Rhinoplasty**: Nose reshaping or septum correction is among the most popular procedures, often driven by facial symmetry or proportion dissatisfaction.
- **Chin Enhancement**: Often combined with rhinoplasty to achieve a balanced profile.
- **Breast Reduction**: Performed to alleviate physical discomfort, such as back or neck pain, or to improve self-esteem.
- **Correction of Breast Asymmetry**: A procedure to balance uneven breast sizes, particularly common during adolescence when breasts develop at different rates.
- **Labiaplasty**: Reduction or reshaping of the labia minora, often sought for aesthetic reasons or to reduce discomfort during physical activity.

- **Scar and Blemish Removal**: Procedures to minimize the appearance of acne scars or other skin imperfections, reflecting the high prevalence of acne among adolescents.

Social media plays a significant role in shaping teenagers' perceptions of beauty and self-worth. Platforms like Instagram and TikTok are flooded with images of "perfect" faces and bodies, often edited or filtered, setting unrealistic beauty standards. Teenagers, already vulnerable to peer pressure, may internalize these standards and feel compelled to conform.

Furthermore, celebrities and influencers openly discussing their cosmetic procedures contribute to the normalization of plastic surgery among young people. The constant exposure to these idealized images can intensify feelings of inadequacy and amplify the desire for surgical solutions.

Many teenagers approach plastic surgery with unrealistic expectations, believing it will solve all their problems or drastically improve their social relationships. However, altering one's appearance is unlikely to result in increased love, acceptance, or validation from others.

Plastic surgery also carries risks, including:

- **Complications**: Infections, scarring, or asymmetrical results.
- **Regret**: Dissatisfaction with the outcome, mainly as the body grows and changes during adolescence.
- **Psychological Impact**: Surgery can reinforce insecurities rather than resolve them, mainly if the cause of dissatisfaction is deeper self-esteem issues.

In most cases, adolescents do not truly need plastic surgery. Many perceived flaws resolve naturally over time as the body matures, and self-confidence grows. For example, facial features such as the nose and chin continue to develop into early adulthood, and hormonal changes often improve skin texture and tone.

Reputable plastic surgeons often recommend that teenagers undergo psychological evaluation before committing to surgery. A psychologist can help identify whether the desire for surgery stems from social pressure, bullying, or an underlying mental health concern, such as body dysmorphic disorder (BDD).

Parents, educators, and healthcare providers play crucial roles in guiding teenagers through this critical stage of self-discovery. Encouraging teens to focus on self-acceptance, healthy habits, and building confidence in their natural beauty often mitigates the desire for surgical interventions.

Engaging in activities that promote self-esteem, such as sports, the arts, or volunteering, can shift the focus away from physical appearance and help adolescents develop a sense of worth beyond their looks. Open conversations about the unrealistic standards perpetuated by social media and the importance of individuality can also empower teens to embrace their unique qualities.

Parents and mentors can help teenagers navigate this period without resorting to unnecessary and potentially harmful surgical solutions by fostering a supportive environment and emphasizing inner strengths.

Did You Know?

- *Over 80% of teenage girls are influenced by societal beauty standards, often leading them to experiment with makeup or consider altering their appearance to fit these ideals.*
- *Nearly 300,000 teenagers in the U.S. undergo plastic surgery each year, with rhinoplasty and breast reduction being among the most popular procedures.*

Tattoos: Expression, Art, and Considerations

Once stigmatized as symbols of rebellion or criminal affiliation, tattoos have evolved into a widely accepted form of body art and self-expression. Today, tattoos are commonplace and embraced by people of all ages, professions, and even entire families. From minimalistic designs to intricate works of art, tattoos have become a way for individuals to tell their stories, memorialize essential moments, or adorn their bodies with beauty.

Tattoos, however, are not merely decorative; they are a permanent modification to the body, and the decision to get one requires careful thought, especially for teenagers. Understanding the process, the risks, and the potential for regret can help ensure a positive and informed experience.

A tattoo is a deliberate injury to the skin. Ink is injected into the dermis, the deeper layer of skin beneath the epidermis. Unlike the epidermis, which regenerates regularly, the dermis holds the ink permanently, giving tattoos their lasting nature. Tattooing is typically performed using specialized machines that ensure precision and safety by controlling the depth of needle penetration, usually no deeper than 1–2 millimeters.

The time required for a tattoo depends on its size, complexity, and technique. Some designs are completed in minutes, while others may take hours or multiple sessions spread over days or weeks.

What Should Teens and Parents Know Before Getting a Tattoo?

- **Tattooing Is a Medical Procedure:**

A tattoo breaks the skin barrier, creating an open wound requiring care to prevent infection. Swelling, redness, and pain are common immediately after tattooing, and the risk of infection increases significantly without proper aftercare.

- **Sterile Conditions Are Essential:**

Ensure the tattoo studio follows strict hygiene protocols. Needles must be disposable and sterile, and artists should wear gloves and masks. The studio should also have an autoclave for sterilizing reusable equipment.

- **Health Conditions to Consider:**

Tattoos may not be suitable for individuals with certain conditions, including:

•

- Cardiovascular diseases
- Diabetes
- Skin disorders like eczema or psoriasis
- Blood clotting disorders
- Allergies to tattoo ink

Teens considering tattoos should consult a healthcare provider if they have any underlying medical conditions.

❖ **Vaccination:**

Ensure vaccinations for hepatitis B and tetanus are up-to-date before getting a tattoo.

❖ **Long-Term Commitment:**

A tattoo is a permanent mark, so teens must consider its impact on future career opportunities and personal preferences. While more accepted today, visible tattoos may still be frowned upon in certain professions.

❖ **Pain and Healing:**

The tattooing process can be painful, especially in sensitive areas like ribs or feet. Healing takes 2–4 weeks, during which time the tattoo must be kept clean, moisturized, and protected from sunlight.

Proper aftercare is crucial for preventing infections and ensuring the tattoo heals well. Here are some tips:

- Keep the tattoo covered with a sterile bandage for the first 24 hours.
- Wash the tattoo with mild soap and water, patting it dry with a clean towel.
- Apply a thin layer of fragrance-free moisturizer or a recommended tattoo ointment.
- Avoid direct sunlight, swimming, and activities that cause excessive sweating during the healing process.
- Do not pick at scabs or peeling skin, as this can cause scarring or uneven ink retention.

Despite the growing popularity of tattoos, regret is not uncommon. Surveys indicate that nearly 25% of people with tattoos consider removing at least one. The reasons vary - shifts in personal style, professional constraints, or the fading quality of older tattoos.

1. **Laser Tattoo Removal:**

Laser removal is the most common method. High-intensity laser beams break down ink particles, which the body eliminates through natural processes. Depending on the size, color, and age of the tattoo, multiple sessions are often required.

- Advantages: Effective on most tattoos and minimally invasive.
- Disadvantages**:** It is painful, expensive, and may not completely remove the tattoo. Some colors, like green and yellow, are harder to erase.

2. **Dermabrasion:**

This method involves sanding down the skin's surface to remove the tattoo.

- Advantages: You can remove tattoos in fewer sessions.
- Disadvantages**:** Highly invasive, painful, and carries a risk of scarring.

3. **Surgical Removal:**

Small tattoos can be excised surgically.

- Advantages: Completely removes the tattoo in one procedure.
- Disadvantages**:** Only suitable for small tattoos; leaves a scar.

4. **Tattoo Cover-Ups:**

Some opt for a cover-up design rather than removing a tattoo. A skilled artist can incorporate the old tattoo into a new, more desirable one.

- Advantages: Less painful and costly than removal.
- Disadvantages: Limited by the size and color of the existing tattoo.

For teens, tattoos can represent a rite of passage or a way to assert individuality. However, adolescence's impulsivity can lead to rushed decisions. Parents should maintain open communication, emphasizing that tattoos are permanent and encouraging teens to think long-term about their choices.

Teenagers often face peer pressure or are influenced by trends. Discussing the motivations behind wanting a tattoo can help teens make more thoughtful decisions. For example, are they getting tattoos to express personal values or to fit in with a group? Specific tattoo designs—cultural or religious symbols—carry more profound significance. Teens should be encouraged to research the origins and meanings of their chosen designs to avoid cultural appropriation or unintended offense.

Tattoos can be a meaningful form of self-expression, but they require careful consideration, especially for teenagers. Parents can help their teens make informed and responsible choices by fostering open communication and providing education about the process, risks, and long-term implications. If a teen decides to get a tattoo, ensuring they choose a reputable artist and follow proper aftercare guidelines will make the experience safer and more positive.

Tattoo removal is always an option, but it is costly, time-consuming, and not guaranteed to restore the skin thoroughly. Encouraging teens to take their time and consider all aspects before getting inked can help minimize regret and ensure their decision reflects their true values and intentions.

Piercing: A Blend of Tradition, Fashion, and Risks

Piercing involves creating a hole or opening in the skin or other body parts to insert jewelry. While ear piercing for earrings is often considered a harmless cultural or familial tradition, piercing other areas of the body has historically faced societal resistance. In many cultures, baby girls have their earlobes pierced shortly after birth as a rite of passage or aesthetic custom. However, piercings beyond the earlobes, such as those on the nose, lips, tongue, or navel, were once associated with rebellion or unconventional lifestyles.

Over the past two decades, piercing has gained significant mainstream popularity, becoming a widely accepted form of self-expression, fashion, and even spirituality. For some, piercings carry cultural or religious significance, while others represent individuality or alignment with current trends.

Despite its growing acceptance, piercing is not a decision to be taken lightly. It involves medical and aesthetic considerations, particularly for teenagers who may be drawn to it to assert independence or fit in with their peers.

Although piercing is a common practice, it is far from risk-free. It involves breaking the skin barrier, making it an invasive procedure. Potential risks include:

- **Infections**: Bacterial infections are the most common complication, especially when proper aftercare or hygiene is neglected.
- **Bleeding**: Improper technique or piercing through highly vascularized areas can lead to excessive bleeding.
- **Scarring**: Improper healing may result in noticeable scars.
- **Keloid Formation**: Some individuals are prone to keloids — raised, overgrown scars that can be painful and unsightly.

Teenagers often choose to pierce visible areas like the nose, lips, tongue, eyebrows, and navel or intimate areas such as the nipples or genitals. While visible piercings are often intended to make a statement or attract attention, intimate piercings are sometimes linked to enhanced sexual pleasure. However, these piercings carry higher risks of discomfort, infection, and inflammation due to the sensitive nature of the skin and mucous membranes in these areas.

It is estimated that around 13% of teenagers have piercings their parents are unaware of, often due to fear of disapproval or restriction. This secrecy increases the likelihood of unsafe procedures performed by untrained individuals, amplifying the risk of complications.

What Parents and Teens Should Know About Piercing

As with tattoos, some countries regulate piercing, allowing it only for individuals over 18 or requiring parental consent for minors. Legal restrictions, however, sometimes drive teenagers to seek out unregulated or do-it-yourself (DIY) piercings, which significantly increase health risks.

Parents should maintain open communication rather than dismiss or forbid a teen's desire for a piercing. By understanding their child's motivations and guiding them toward safe practices, parents can ensure that the decision is made responsibly and safely.

Piercing must be performed under professional, sterile conditions to minimize risks and ensure proper healing. Here are essential safety measures:

1. **Choose a Licensed Professional**:
    - Verify the piercer's credentials and ensure they work in a licensed facility.
    - Visit the studio beforehand to assess cleanliness, proper sterilization techniques, and adherence to hygiene standards.
2. **Ensure Sterile Tools**:
    - Needles must be single-use and sterile.
    - The piercer should wear disposable gloves, which must be changed between clients.
3. **Vaccination Is Key**:
    - Teens should be vaccinated against hepatitis B and tetanus before undergoing any piercing procedure.
4. **Understand Healing Times**:
    - Earlobes: Typically heal in 4–6 weeks.
    - Cartilage (upper ear): Can take 4–12 months.
    - Navel: Healing may take 6 months to a year and is prone to irritation from clothing.
    - Nose: Heals in 2–4 months, but infection risks are higher due to bacteria in the nasal cavity.
    - Tongue and Lips: Heal relatively quickly (4–6 weeks), but risks include swelling, speech difficulties, and tooth damage.
    - Genital Piercings: Require meticulous hygiene and can take months to heal, with frequent risks of infection and inflammation.

Teenagers and parents should also consider the social implications of visible piercings. Some schools, workplaces, and extracurricular programs prohibit visible piercings or enforce dress codes restricting their use. Understanding these restrictions in advance can prevent conflicts or misunderstandings.

Additionally, cultural norms around piercings vary widely. In some traditions, nose piercings or earrings signify marital status or community belonging, while in others, they are purely aesthetic. Teens should be encouraged to understand the cultural or symbolic meaning behind their chosen piercings to ensure their decisions are respectful and well-informed.

Proper aftercare is critical to prevent infections and promote healing. General aftercare guidelines include:

1. Clean the piercing site twice daily with a saline solution or an antiseptic recommended by the piercer.
2. Avoid touching the piercing with unwashed hands.
3. Do not remove or change the jewelry until the piercing has healed completely.
4. Avoid swimming in pools, hot tubs, or natural bodies of water during healing.
5. Opt for loose clothing or avoid friction near body piercings like the navel or genitals.

If signs of infection occur, such as redness, swelling, excessive pain, discharge, or fever, consult a healthcare provider promptly.

While piercings are less permanent than tattoos, many people eventually remove them. This is particularly common for piercings in sensitive areas, like the nose, tongue, or genitals, due to:

- Persistent discomfort or pain.
- Irritation from jewelry.
- Frequent inflammation or infections.
- Changes in personal or professional circumstances.

If jewelry is removed, the piercing hole may close independently, depending on the location and how long it has been in place. However, scar tissue often remains, especially in larger or stretched piercings.

For individuals who regret their piercings, removal is straightforward in most cases. The jewelry is removed, and the hole can heal naturally. However, the extent of healing depends on the piercing's location and how long it has been there.

- Small Piercings (e.g., earlobes) often close wholly within weeks or months.
- Cartilage Piercings: May not close entirely, leaving a slight indentation or scar.
- Stretched Piercings (e.g., gauges): Require surgical correction to repair the stretched skin.

For teens considering piercings, emphasizing the potential for scarring or incomplete healing can encourage them to think carefully before proceeding.

Piercing can be an exciting form of self-expression, but it comes with medical, social, and long-term considerations. By fostering open discussions and educating teens about the risks, aftercare, and possible outcomes, parents can guide them toward making informed and responsible choices. Whether it's a simple earlobe piercing or something more elaborate, prioritizing safety and hygiene ensures a positive experience.

Did You Know?

- *Nearly 25% of tattooed individuals consider removing at least one tattoo later in life, often due to changes in personal style or professional requirements.*
- *Around 13% of teenagers have piercings that their parents are unaware of, increasing the risk of complications from unsafe, unregulated procedures.*

Sports and a Girl's Health

Sports and physical activity significantly shape a girl's physical, emotional, and mental well-being. However, they also bring unique challenges during adolescence, when the body undergoes significant hormonal and developmental changes. Balancing the benefits of physical activity with the demands of growing up is key to ensuring long-term health and happiness.

Adolescence is often a period of exploration, and for many girls, sports become a meaningful outlet for self-expression, fitness, and social interaction. While some girls embrace sports willingly, drawn by the joy of physical activity and camaraderie, others are pushed into athletic pursuits by parents eager to fulfill their unrealized dreams. In such cases, sports can lose their inherent joy, becoming a burden rather than a source of pleasure.

Parents' intentions are often well-meaning; they see sports to instill discipline, build character, and foster resilience. However, in some families, children spend every day after school juggling intense training schedules and extracurricular activities, leaving little time for rest or hobbies. This over-scheduling can deprive them of the carefree nature of childhood, making physical activity feel more like an obligation than an enjoyable pursuit.

Physical activity is undoubtedly beneficial, but it can strain the body when it becomes excessive or poorly managed. Competitive sports often impose demands that conflict with what is medically advisable for growing adolescents. This is especially true in sports that prioritize low body weight or specific body types, where athletes may be encouraged to maintain extremely low weight-to-height ratios.

For some adolescent athletes, the consequences of overtraining include chronic fatigue, disrupted sleep patterns, loss of appetite, and even mood disturbances. In extreme cases, this imbalance can lead to long-term physical and emotional health challenges.

Puberty is a transformative phase in a girl's life, and regular menstrual cycles are a critical marker of her hormonal and reproductive health. Intense physical training, however, can disrupt this delicate balance in several ways. High physical activity levels can delay menarche, the first menstrual period, or lead to irregular cycles. These disruptions are often tied to insufficient body fat, essential for producing sex hormones like estrogen and progesterone.

A particularly concerning condition seen in adolescent athletes is the **Female Athlete Triad**. This syndrome, common among girls engaged in rigorous sports, consists of three interconnected issues:

1. **Energy Deficiency**: When caloric intake fails to meet the body's energy demands, an imbalance can result, impacting overall health.
2. **Menstrual Dysfunction**: Irregular or absent menstrual cycles often result from hormonal disruptions caused by inadequate nutrition and overtraining.
3. **Decreased Bone Mineral Density**: Without sufficient estrogen levels, bones lose density, increasing the risk of fractures and conditions like osteoporosis.

The triad underscores the importance of balancing physical activity with proper nutrition, adequate rest, and regular health monitoring. Encouraging girls to approach sports as a source of joy and personal growth rather than purely as a means of achieving competitive success can help prevent these health challenges.

Proper nutrition is the cornerstone of athletic performance and overall health, yet adolescent athletes, their parents, and even their coaches often overlook or misunderstand. Girls in weight-sensitive sports may fear gaining weight, leading to inadequate caloric intake. Others may consume normal food portions but find that intense physical activity still leaves them with an energy deficit.

When the body lacks the energy and nutrients it needs, it prioritizes vital functions over reproduction, resulting in hormonal imbalances and disrupted menstrual cycles. **Amenorrhea**, or the absence of menstruation for six months or more, is a common consequence of poor nutrition and excessive physical activity. While irregular cycles are regular during the early stages of adolescence, prolonged amenorrhea is a serious health concern that warrants medical attention.

Contrary to the assumption that sports constantly strengthen bones, hormonal imbalances caused by overtraining can hinder calcium metabolism. Estrogen is crucial in maintaining bone density; irregular menstrual cycles disrupt this process. As a result, adolescent athletes with infrequent or absent periods may experience bone loss, similar to what is seen in postmenopausal women. Monitoring bone density and addressing any signs of menstrual irregularities are critical to preventing long-term complications.

The menstrual cycle itself can influence athletic performance. During the first phase of the cycle, many girls feel more energetic and perform better in physical activities. In contrast, the days leading up to menstruation are often marked by fatigue, abdominal discomfort, and a general decrease in energy levels. Some coaches recommend using hormonal contraceptives to regulate or delay menstruation during competitions. Still, this approach is not always suitable for younger girls and should be carefully evaluated on a case-by-case basis.

While it is generally safe for girls to remain physically active during menstruation, certain adjustments may be necessary. For example, intense exercises targeting the lower abdomen should be avoided, especially during the first few days of menstruation, as they may exacerbate discomfort. Theories suggesting a link between strenuous activity during menstruation and conditions like endometriosis remain unproven, but moderate activity is widely considered safe and beneficial.

At the other end of the spectrum, a sedentary lifestyle poses its risks, including obesity and related health issues such as diabetes and cardiovascular disease. Childhood and adolescent obesity are on the rise in many countries, underscoring the importance of promoting balanced nutrition and regular physical activity from an early age.

Preventing obesity requires a multifaceted approach, including education about healthy eating habits, encouragement of consistent physical activity, and fostering a balanced lifestyle that integrates exercise, rest, and proper nutrition.

Adolescent girls' sports should be about more than competition; they should be a pathway to physical fitness, personal growth, and enjoyment. Striking a balance between activity, nutrition, and rest is essential for safeguarding their immediate and long-term health. Parents, coaches, and healthcare providers can help young athletes thrive in every aspect of their lives by fostering a supportive environment and prioritizing well-being over performance metrics.

Did You Know?

- *The Female Athlete Triad—energy deficiency, menstrual dysfunction, and decreased bone density—is a common yet preventable condition among adolescent athletes, highlighting the need for balanced nutrition and rest.*
- *Amenorrhea in adolescent athletes can signal underlying health issues, such as hormonal imbalances or inadequate nutrition, and should not be ignored.*

Bad Habits and Adolescents

Adolescence is a time of exploration and identity formation, but it's also a period of heightened vulnerability to negative influences. Children and teenagers often imitate the behavior of adults around them, especially those they admire or see as role models. This is why many young people admit to experimenting with smoking or alcohol at surprisingly young ages, sometimes as early as 8, 10, or 12. Unfortunately, these introductions often happen within the home, during family gatherings, where adults casually offer champagne or condone a taste of beer, unknowingly setting a precedent. Peer pressure also plays a significant role, but the family environment remains among the earliest and most influential factors.

Smoking

Smoking is not just a habit; for many adolescents, it represents rebellion, independence, and maturity. Smoking often appears glamorous due to its portrayal in popular culture, with celebrities and influencers frequently depicted smoking. Among adolescent girls, smoking is sometimes used to reject traditional "good girl" stereotypes and embrace a "bad girl" image, one that is rebellious, carefree, and bold. Boys often associate smoking with masculinity, toughness, or peer acceptance.

Despite its allure, smoking is a leading cause of preventable illness and death. Adolescents, however, often dismiss these risks, as the harmful effects of smoking do not manifest immediately.

- Around 20% of adolescents smoke, with significant variation across regions.
- More than 30% of children start smoking by age 12 or earlier.
- Approximately 60% of adolescents first try smoking with friends, while 10% are introduced to it by family members.

- 60% of smoking adolescents have at least one family member who smokes, highlighting the strong influence of household environments.
- Among adolescents aged 15 and under, 15% of girls and 16% of boys are smokers. By late adolescence, these numbers increase to 20% for girls and 30% for boys.

The landscape of smoking has shifted dramatically over the past two decades. While traditional cigarettes remain common, many teens now experiment with cigars, pipes, and particularly hookah, which is often falsely perceived as less harmful.

The rise of electronic cigarettes (e-cigarettes) has also been staggering, with high school students being the largest group of users. The legalization of medical marijuana in various countries has further complicated the issue, as some adolescents misuse it recreationally, often combining it with smoking.

These alternatives, though marketed as safer, carry their health risks. Hookah smoke, for example, contains toxic substances at levels often higher than those in cigarette smoke, while e-cigarettes may contain harmful chemicals and lead to nicotine addiction.

Adolescents who smoke are significantly more likely to engage in other risky behaviors, including:

- Alcohol and drug use, particularly cocaine.
- Aggression and physical altercations.
- Carrying firearms or engaging in violence.
- Suicide attempts.
- Mental health issues such as depression and anxiety.
- Unsafe sexual practices increase the risk of sexually transmitted infections (STIs) and unplanned pregnancies.

Efforts to curb smoking through public awareness campaigns and stricter regulations have reduced smoking rates among adolescents in many developed countries, but the broader behavioral and psychological consequences of smoking remain a critical challenge.

One of the reasons adolescents underestimate the dangers of smoking is its delayed impact. The adverse effects often become evident only years or decades later, fostering a false sense of security. However, it is crucial to communicate to adolescents that smokers, on average, live 13–14 years less than non-smokers.

Smoking is a major contributor to diseases such as cardiovascular conditions, lung cancer, and other forms of cancer. Among adolescent girls, smoking has specific implications for reproductive health. While research is still emerging, prolonged smoking is known to affect menstrual cycles and the maturation of reproductive cells. It increases the risk of precancerous conditions and cervical cancer, especially when combined with other risk factors such as human papillomavirus (HPV) infection.

Quitting smoking is particularly difficult for adolescents, whose impulsive and emotionally driven behavior often overrides rational decision-making. Social circles play a pivotal role; adolescents who spend time with smokers are far less likely to quit. For many, quitting is not just a matter of willpower but also a psychological and social challenge.

Numerous smoking cessation programs cater specifically to teenagers. These programs emphasize psychological support, which significantly increases the likelihood of success. Techniques such as counseling, behavioral therapy, and nicotine replacement options can help, but sustained support from family and peers is essential for lasting change.

Addressing smoking among adolescents requires a comprehensive strategy that includes education, support, and prevention. Stricter smoking regulations in public places, combined with accessible education campaigns, have successfully reduced adolescent smoking rates in many countries by up to 50% over the last decade. However, these efforts must also tackle the broader behavioral patterns associated with smoking to ensure adolescents are equipped to make informed, health-conscious choices.

Families and communities can help adolescents navigate this challenging phase and avoid the long-term consequences of harmful habits by fostering open communication, providing resources for cessation, and modeling healthy behaviors.

Alcohol

Adolescents often perceive alcohol as a gateway to adulthood, a chance to emulate the "forbidden" behaviors they observe in adults. The allure of alcohol is compounded by its normalization in many households, where parents might casually allow children a sip during family celebrations. For some teens, the first experience with alcohol happens under peer pressure, while for others, it begins at home, with seemingly harmless gestures that pave the way for future habits.

Studies reveal that alcohol consumption among adolescents is a pervasive issue worldwide. In the United States, over 50% of individuals aged 12–20 have tried alcohol, and in many developed nations, the average age of first consumption is 11 years for boys and 13 years for girls. These statistics highlight the urgency of addressing the factors that lead to early alcohol exposure.

Adolescents who consume alcohol are significantly more likely to engage in risky and destructive behaviors, including:

- **Aggressive behavior**: Alcohol lowers inhibitions, often leading to confrontations or violent outbursts.
- **Criminal activities**: Theft, vandalism, and even assault are more common among teens who drink.
- **Risky sexual behavior**: Alcohol impairs judgment, increasing the likelihood of unprotected sex and multiple partners, often leading to sexually transmitted infections (STIs) or unplanned pregnancies.
- **Alcohol addiction in adulthood**: Early exposure and habitual use during adolescence significantly increase the risk of dependency later in life.

Adolescent girls who consume alcohol are particularly vulnerable to becoming victims of physical and sexual violence, making the consequences of drinking even more severe for them. Several factors contribute to why some adolescents are more likely to experiment with or regularly consume alcohol. These include:

- **Family influence**: Adolescents with parents or siblings who drink heavily are more likely to follow suit.

- **Peer pressure**: Friends often introduce teens to alcohol, creating a social environment where drinking is normalized.
- **Mental health issues**: Depression, anxiety, anger dysregulation, and schizophrenia increase vulnerability to alcohol use.
- **Genetic predisposition**: A family history of alcoholism raises the likelihood of dependency.
- **Socioeconomic and cultural background**: Alcohol use varies across ethnic and racial groups, with some communities experiencing higher rates of consumption.
- **Gender differences**: While boys consume larger quantities of alcohol, girls tend to develop dependence more quickly and with smaller amounts.

Alcohol use is particularly prevalent among high school and university students across many countries. Former Soviet republics report some of the highest rates of alcohol consumption among youth. In the United States, 50% of high school seniors consume alcohol, and over 14% have experienced significant intoxication at least once a year. Approximately 8% of teens report binge drinking, consuming multiple shots of hard liquor in one sitting.

These figures underscore the need for comprehensive strategies to curb adolescent alcohol use.

Alcohol addiction often progresses through identifiable stages. Recognizing these stages can help parents, educators, and healthcare providers intervene early:

1. **Initial Exposure**: Alcohol is often viewed as a low-risk substance compared to cigarettes or drugs; curiosity, peer pressure, and a desire to fit in drive initial use.
2. **Experimentation**: Drinking becomes a regular activity, often accompanied by smoking or drug use, as teens explore their limits.
3. **Increased Usage**: Consumption frequency and quantity escalate. Adolescents actively seek out alcohol, sometimes resorting to theft or other means to obtain it.

4. **Regular Use and Obsession**: Alcohol becomes central to the teen's life. School performance, family relationships, and social dynamics begin to deteriorate.
5. **Complete Dependency**: At this stage, the adolescent feels normal only when intoxicated. Behavior becomes erratic, and criminal activities may occur to fund their addiction.

Alcohol impairs concentration, memory, and learning, affecting academic performance. Poor nutrition or malnutrition, often associated with adolescent alcoholism, leads to long-term health issues. Driving under the influence is particularly dangerous for adolescents, contributing to 60% of traffic fatalities among individuals aged 15–20. Mental health challenges, including depression, are exacerbated by alcohol use, contributing to higher rates of suicide among teens who drink.

Adolescent girls face unique risks from alcohol consumption:

- Menstrual irregularities: Alcohol disrupts hormonal balance, leading to missed or irregular periods.
- Reproductive health risks: Alcohol increases vulnerability to STIs due to impaired judgment and inconsistent use of protection.
- Unplanned pregnancies: Many intoxicated encounters result in unintended consequences, including pregnancy.

Early and effective prevention is essential to address adolescent alcohol use. One of the most critical steps is providing education about the dangers of alcohol before children reach adolescence. When children understand the potential risks, including health consequences, impaired judgment, and long-term dependency, they are better equipped to make informed decisions. Prevention efforts should begin early and include open discussions at home, in schools, and within communities.

Parental involvement plays a pivotal role in shaping adolescents' attitudes toward alcohol. Parents should engage in honest, judgment-free conversations about alcohol's effects, fostering trust and helping teens feel comfortable discussing their experiences and pressures. By establishing a foundation of open communication, parents can create a supportive environment that discourages alcohol use and promotes healthy coping mechanisms.

Another effective strategy is keeping adolescents engaged in meaningful activities. After-school programs, sports, hobbies, and creative pursuits occupy their time and help build confidence, discipline, and a sense of purpose. These activities provide a constructive outlet for energy and emotions, reducing the likelihood of boredom or peer pressure leading to experimentation with alcohol. Furthermore, sharing relatable real-life stories about the consequences of alcohol use can deeply resonate with teens, making the dangers more tangible and personal.

For adolescents who are already struggling with alcohol use, intervention requires a multifaceted approach. Psychological counseling can address the emotional and social factors driving their behavior, providing tools to manage stress, peer pressure, and underlying mental health issues. Family involvement is equally crucial, as a stable and supportive home environment can significantly influence recovery. In more severe cases, rehabilitation programs may be necessary to break the cycle of dependency, offering structured support and professional care.

Timing and environment also play a significant role in adolescent alcohol consumption. Statistics reveal that the highest incidence of alcohol use occurs between **3:00 PM and 6:00 PM,** a window of unsupervised time when many teens are home from school and parents are not yet home from work. This highlights the importance of structured activities and consistent parental presence during these vulnerable hours. Providing opportunities for engagement, whether through clubs, sports, or community programs, can deter teens from turning to alcohol out of boredom or curiosity.

By combining education, active parental involvement, structured activities, and professional support when needed, families and communities can create a protective framework that helps adolescents navigate the challenges of peer pressure and risky behaviors. These proactive measures not only mitigate the risks of alcohol use but also foster healthier habits and decision-making for the future.

Drugs

Adolescence is a period of exploration and curiosity, but it can also be a time of vulnerability to harmful behaviors. Among these, drug use poses one of the most significant risks, often entangled with smoking and alcohol consumption in a dangerous triad. Adolescents who experiment with one of these habits are statistically more likely to engage in the others, creating a compounding effect on their health and prospects.

Drug addiction is a pervasive issue that transcends borders, affecting individuals from all backgrounds. The global drug trade thrives on secrecy, and the accurate scale of drug use among adolescents is challenging to measure. Public attention often focuses on extreme cases where users end up in hospitals, face legal troubles, or lose their lives.

Adolescents are particularly prone to experimentation, often using substances that are readily available, such as prescription medications, household chemicals, and other accessible items. These substances, while not always classified as drugs, can be equally harmful or even deadly in specific doses. The wide array of substances abused by teenagers reflects a growing problem that requires urgent attention.

Adolescents commonly experiment with a range of substances, including:

- **Traditional drugs**: Cocaine, heroin, crack, amphetamines, marijuana, and hallucinogens like PCP and LSD.
- **Inhalants**: Household products like butane, paint, and glue, which are inexpensive and easily accessible.
- **Medications**: Sedatives, painkillers, and anticonvulsants are often misused for their psychoactive effects.

While traditional drugs remain a concern, the increasing use of inhalants and prescription medications highlights the dangers of substances that may seem harmless or less regulated.

Adolescent drug use exhibits notable gender differences:

- ❖ **Girls**: More likely to misuse medications, often to self-soothe or escape emotional problems. They are also more likely to combine alcohol with drugs, increasing the risk of dependency.
- ❖ **Boys** tend to use traditional drugs, often in social settings, to enhance pleasure or boost confidence.

These patterns underline the need for tailored prevention and intervention strategies that address each gender's unique motivations and risks.

Recent years have seen a rise in marijuana use among adolescent girls and fluctuating trends in the use of substances like Ecstasy (MDMA). A troubling development is the combination of alcohol with medications or non-traditional drugs, as many girls mistakenly believe these combinations are safe.

Interestingly, some high-achieving girls in academics have been found to engage in substance abuse. Peer influence plays a significant role in these behaviors, with close friends who use drugs or alcohol often encouraging similar habits within their social circles.

The consequences of drug abuse extend beyond the individual, impacting families and society. Addiction not only deteriorates physical and mental health but also disrupts relationships, education, and career prospects. Adolescents who abuse drugs are at greater risk of:

- **Health complications**: From poisoning and organ damage to long-term addiction.
- **Mental health issues**, including depression and anxiety, are often exacerbated by substance abuse.
- **Social consequences**: Legal troubles, strained family relationships, and academic failure.

Drug dependency in adolescence rarely resolves without intervention, emphasizing the importance of early detection and action.

Education is the cornerstone of prevention. Parents should teach children about the dangers of drug use early, fostering open and honest discussions about the risks and consequences. Adolescents are more likely to resist peer pressure when they feel informed and supported.

When parents suspect drug use, taking immediate action is critical. Many countries offer free resources and anonymous support programs to educate families about substance abuse and guide them through the recovery process. Contrary to common misconceptions, parents wield significant influence and are often the first line of defense against addiction.

Schools, community organizations, and religious groups often have trained professionals who specialize in addressing substance abuse. These experts can provide counseling and intervention strategies tailored to the adolescent's needs.

Regular, meaningful interactions between parents and adolescents can help prevent and address substance abuse. Trust-based relationships encourage teens to share their struggles and seek help before problems escalate.

Addiction does not happen overnight; it typically follows a progression:

1. **Initial Exposure**: Often motivated by curiosity or peer pressure, adolescents try substances they perceive as less harmful.
2. **Experimentation**: Substances are used occasionally in social settings, with teens testing their limits.
3. **Increased Usage**: Frequency and quantity increase, with adolescents actively seeking substances.
4. **Regular Use and Obsession**: Substance use becomes habitual, overshadowing other aspects of life.
5. **Complete Dependency**: Addiction takes hold, leading to aggressive behavior, isolation, and often criminal activities to fund the habit.

Understanding these stages can help parents and professionals intervene effectively at the earliest signs of substance abuse. Early detection of substance abuse dramatically improves the chances of successful recovery. Parents should remain vigilant for signs of drug use, such as behavioral changes, academic decline, and withdrawal from family and friends. Open communication and timely intervention can make all the difference in preventing the escalation of addiction.

Addressing adolescent drug use requires a collaborative effort among families, schools, and communities. By fostering supportive environments, providing access to resources, and equipping teens with the knowledge to make informed decisions, society can reduce the prevalence of substance abuse and its devastating effects.

Prevention starts with awareness, and intervention begins with understanding. Together, these strategies can help adolescents avoid the dangers of drug use and lead healthier, more fulfilling lives.

Did You Know?

- *Smoking Adolescents Are More Vulnerable to Risky Behaviors: Teens who smoke are significantly more likely to experiment with alcohol, drugs, and unsafe sexual practices, highlighting the interconnected nature of harmful habits.*
- *Adolescent Alcohol Use Peaks Between 3:00 PM and 6:00 PM: Unsupervised hours after school are a critical period for teens, emphasizing the importance of structured activities and parental engagement.*

Mental Health and Emotional Well-Being

Mental health and emotional well-being are foundational to children's overall development and success, shaping their ability to navigate life's challenges, build meaningful relationships, and pursue their aspirations. These aspects are particularly nuanced for girls, influenced by a complex interplay of biological, psychological, social, and cultural factors. While the topic of mental health has gained increased attention in recent years, the unique experiences and needs of girls often remain underexplored in both academic research and public discourse. This chapter seeks to illuminate the critical aspects of girls' mental health and emotional well-being, drawing attention to their developmental trajectories and the challenges they face.

From early childhood through adolescence, girls undergo significant physiological and emotional changes that influence their mental health. Hormonal fluctuations during puberty, coupled with evolving social expectations and pressures, can heighten their vulnerability to mental health challenges. Conditions such as anxiety, depression, and eating disorders often manifest during this period, necessitating early intervention and support. However, mental health is not solely defined by the presence or absence of disorders; it also encompasses resilience, self-esteem, and the ability to regulate emotions. For girls, these qualities are shaped by their immediate family environments and broader societal influences, including media portrayals, gender norms, and peer interactions.

Cultural attitudes toward mental health and gender roles further complicate the picture. In some societies, girls are often discouraged from openly expressing negative emotions, leading to internalized stress and the development of coping mechanisms that may not always be healthy. Conversely, environments that foster open communication, self-expression, and emotional validation can significantly bolster a girl's mental well-being. Thus, understanding the cultural and societal contexts in which girls are raised is essential for creating effective mental health strategies.

The chapter will also delve into the role of caregivers, educators, and healthcare providers in shaping a girl's emotional landscape. Supportive relationships, positive reinforcement, and access to mental health resources play pivotal roles in promoting emotional resilience and mitigating the risks of mental health disorders. Evidence-based practices, such as mindfulness, cognitive-behavioral strategies, and peer support programs, have successfully improved mental health outcomes in girls and will be explored in detail.

Ultimately, this chapter underscores the importance of a holistic approach to girls' mental health and emotional well-being. By addressing the biological, psychological, and social dimensions of mental health, we can better equip girls to thrive in all areas of their lives. In doing so, we not only empower the individual but also lay the groundwork for healthier families and communities, recognizing that the well-being of girls today shapes the future of society tomorrow.

Stress and Anxiety Management

Stress and anxiety are universal human experiences, yet they manifest uniquely in girls due to the interplay of biological, psychological, and sociocultural factors. For girls, particularly during formative years, stress can stem from academic pressures, peer relationships, familial expectations, and societal norms that shape their self-perception and sense of worth. Left unaddressed, chronic stress and anxiety can hinder emotional development, compromise mental health, and limit a girl's ability to reach her full potential. Thus, equipping girls with effective resilience and coping strategies is a preventative and empowering measure.

Stress and anxiety often emerge as natural responses to challenges or perceived threats. For girls, these responses may be exacerbated by hormonal changes during puberty, heightened sensitivity to social dynamics, and the pressure to meet cultural expectations of femininity. Academic demands and extracurricular activities can further amplify these stressors, creating a delicate balance between striving for excellence and maintaining emotional health.

Girls also tend to internalize stress differently than boys. While boys may express stress outwardly through disruptive behavior, girls often channel their stress inwardly, which can manifest as anxiety, perfectionism, or self-doubt. This internalization can make their struggles less visible, leading to delayed recognition and intervention. Furthermore, the societal stigma surrounding mental health often discourages girls from seeking help or expressing their emotions openly. These factors highlight the urgent need for proactive approaches that teach girls to recognize, manage, and ultimately overcome stress and anxiety.

Resilience is the ability to adapt and thrive in the face of adversity. Teaching resilience is foundational to helping girls manage stress effectively. Resilience-building fosters a growth mindset, where challenges are viewed as opportunities for learning and personal development rather than insurmountable obstacles. Parents, educators, and caregivers play a pivotal role in modeling resilience and encouraging girls to adopt similar attitudes.

A core component of resilience is **self-awareness**. Encouraging girls to identify their stress triggers and understand their emotional responses is a critical first step. Journaling, mood tracking, and open emotional discussions can help girls develop this awareness. For instance, a girl who recognizes that she feels anxious before public speaking can learn to address this specific fear through targeted strategies, such as visualization or practicing calming techniques.

Another essential element of resilience is fostering a sense of **self-efficacy**. When girls believe in their ability to influence outcomes and navigate challenges, they are less likely to feel overwhelmed by stress. Activities that build competence through sports, academics, or creative pursuits can bolster this belief. Celebrating small successes and reinforcing effort over results further strengthens a girl's confidence in her capabilities.

While resilience provides the foundation, coping strategies offer practical tools for managing stress and anxiety in real time. These strategies should be tailored to a girl's needs and preferences, ensuring they are accessible and sustainable.

- **Mindfulness and Relaxation Techniques**:

Mindfulness practices, such as deep breathing, progressive muscle relaxation, and meditation, can significantly reduce stress levels by grounding girls in the present moment. Teaching mindfulness in accessible formats—such as guided audio sessions or apps—makes these techniques more engaging. Yoga and other movement-based mindfulness activities also combine physical and emotional benefits, promoting relaxation while enhancing body awareness.

- **Cognitive-Behavioral Strategies**:

Cognitive-behavioral techniques empower girls to reframe negative thought patterns and challenge irrational fears. For example, a girl anxious about failing an exam can be guided to replace catastrophic thoughts ("I'll fail everything and disappoint everyone") with constructive ones ("I can prepare effectively, and this is just one test among many"). Teaching girls to identify and counter cognitive distortions cultivates a healthier perspective and reduces anxiety.

- **Time Management and Prioritization**:

A significant source of stress for girls is feeling overwhelmed by responsibilities. Teaching practical skills, such as creating to-do lists, breaking tasks into manageable steps, and setting realistic goals, can alleviate this burden. Introducing girls to concepts like prioritization and the "80/20 rule" helps them focus on what truly matters, reducing unnecessary stress.

- **Social Support and Communication**:

It is vital to encourage girls to seek support from trusted friends, family members, or mentors. Social connections provide emotional validation and practical advice, creating a buffer against stress. Role-playing exercises and assertiveness training can further enhance their ability to communicate needs and set boundaries effectively.

- **Creative Outlets**:

Activities such as drawing, writing, or playing music offer therapeutic benefits by providing an outlet for self-expression. Encouraging girls to explore creative hobbies relieves stress and fosters a sense of accomplishment and joy.

Stress management and resilience-building cannot occur in isolation. Girls thrive in environments that validate their emotions, celebrate their strengths, and provide security. Schools can play a transformative role by incorporating social-emotional learning (SEL) into curricula, equipping girls with lifelong skills for managing emotions and building relationships. Families, too, can contribute by maintaining open lines of communication, modeling healthy coping behaviors, and prioritizing mental health discussions.

Additionally, societal narratives must shift to promote realistic expectations and celebrate individuality. Campaigns that challenge perfectionism and advocate for self-compassion can help girls internalize that it is okay to make mistakes and prioritize their well-being over external validation.

Stress and anxiety are inevitable aspects of life, but they do not have to define a girl's experiences or limit her potential.

We empower girls to navigate challenges confidently and gracefully by teaching resilience and providing effective coping strategies. This empowerment extends beyond individual well-being, fostering a generation of emotionally intense women who are self-aware and equipped to lead fulfilling lives. As caregivers, educators, and advocates, our collective responsibility is to ensure that every girl has the tools and support to thrive, regardless of the obstacles she may encounter.

Building Self-Esteem and Body Image

Self-esteem and body image are critical to a girl's mental and emotional well-being. How a girl perceives herself shapes her confidence, relationships, and ability to navigate life's challenges. However, the modern landscape, marked by pervasive media portrayals and societal expectations, presents unique challenges to developing a positive sense of self. While eating disorders are addressed comprehensively in other chapters, this section focuses on fostering self-esteem and promoting a healthy body image by critically examining external influences and empowering girls with tools for self-acceptance.

In its many forms, media plays a profound role in shaping perceptions of beauty and self-worth. From advertisements and social media influencers to films and television shows, the images girls consume often promote narrow and unrealistic beauty standards. These portrayals frequently emphasize unattainable ideals, such as flawless skin, specific body shapes, and heavily edited features, which can contribute to feelings of inadequacy and dissatisfaction with one's appearance.

For girls, these pressures are magnified by societal expectations that link physical attractiveness to worthiness and success. Cultural norms often place disproportionate emphasis on appearance, encouraging girls to conform to standards that may conflict with their natural diversity. This emphasis distorts body image and detracts from developing other aspects of identity, such as intelligence, creativity, and kindness. Furthermore, social media has amplified these challenges, with platforms providing constant comparisons and validation through likes, comments, and shares.

Self-esteem encompasses a girl's sense of value and confidence in her abilities. Fostering healthy self-esteem begins with helping girls recognize their inherent worth beyond appearance. This involves creating environments prioritizing respect, kindness, and individuality over superficial success metrics.

One of the most effective ways to build self-esteem is by teaching girls to practice positive self-talk. Girls often internalize critical voices, comparing themselves unfavorably to others or focusing on perceived flaws. Encouraging them to challenge these negative thoughts and replace them with affirming statements ("I am capable," "My body is strong and unique") can significantly improve their self-perception. Journaling or using affirmation cards can make this practice more engaging and habitual.

It is vital to help girls embrace their unique qualities, whether physical, intellectual, or emotional. Parents, educators, and mentors can play a pivotal role by highlighting each girl's strengths and talents. For instance, celebrating achievements in academics, sports, or creative pursuits shifts the focus away from appearance and reinforces the idea that self-worth is multifaceted. Introducing girls to diverse role models who exemplify confidence and authenticity can inspire them to embrace their individuality. These role models may come from various backgrounds, professions, and life experiences, illustrating that success and happiness are not tied to conforming to societal norms.

Body image refers to how a girl perceives and feels about her physical self. Cultivating a healthy body image requires dismantling harmful stereotypes and encouraging an appreciation for body diversity.

Teaching girls to analyze media messages critically is a powerful tool for countering negative influences. By deconstructing advertisements, social media posts, and entertainment content, girls can learn to identify manipulation techniques such as photo editing, selective presentation, and unrealistic standards. Discussions about the motives behind these portrayals, such as profit-driven industries, can help girls view media more discerningly.

While eating disorders are discussed in another chapter, it is essential to foster a balanced approach to food and physical activity. Emphasizing the role of nutrition and exercise in promoting health and well-being, rather than appearance, can shift the focus away from weight or aesthetics. This approach reduces the risk of harmful behaviors and reinforces a positive relationship with one's body.

Conversations about societal expectations surrounding beauty should encourage girls to question and redefine these norms. By highlighting beauty standards' historical and cultural variability, girls can better understand that these ideals are arbitrary and ever-changing. Empowering them to set their definitions of beauty promotes autonomy and self-respect.

Girls thrive in environments that validate their experiences and nurture their growth. Families, schools, and communities play a collective role in fostering self-esteem and positive body image. Parents and caregivers should model healthy behaviors, avoid critical comments about appearance, and emphasize unconditional love and acceptance. Schools can incorporate social-emotional learning programs that address self-esteem and media literacy, equipping girls with tools to navigate societal pressures. Community initiatives that celebrate diversity and challenge stereotypes further reinforce these messages.

Building self-esteem and promoting a healthy body image in girls is a multifaceted effort that requires addressing media influences, societal expectations, and individual beliefs. By equipping girls with critical thinking skills, fostering self-acceptance, and creating supportive environments, we empower them to develop a resilient sense of self. Girls are better prepared to challenge external pressures and embrace their full potential as they learn to appreciate their inherent worth and unique qualities. Through these efforts, we lay the foundation for a generation of confident, self-assured women who define beauty and success on their terms.

Screen Time and Social Media: Balancing Online and Offline Life

The digital age has transformed how children, including girls, interact with the world. Technology has become an integral part of daily life, from social media platforms to educational apps. While digital tools offer opportunities for learning, connection, and self-expression, excessive screen time and unbalanced engagement with social media can have detrimental effects on mental health and well-being. This section focuses on strategies to balance online and offline life for girls, emphasizing the importance of mindful technology use. Issues such as cyberbullying and cyberviolence are discussed in greater detail in other chapters.

For many girls, screens represent a gateway to social connection, creativity, and entertainment. Social media platforms provide a space for self-expression and peer interaction. However, these digital interactions can come at a cost. Excessive screen time often replaces essential offline activities, such as physical play, face-to-face conversations, and adequate rest. Furthermore, social media can contribute to anxiety, comparison, and a distorted sense of reality due to curated and idealized portrayals of life.

Girls are particularly vulnerable to social media pressures. The validation-seeking nature of likes, comments, and shares can create a dependence on external approval, leading to lowered self-esteem and increased stress. Additionally, the fear of missing out (FOMO) often compels girls to spend prolonged hours online, disrupting their daily routines and hindering their ability to focus on offline priorities.

Balancing online and offline life requires intentional strategies encouraging girls to use technology in moderation while prioritizing meaningful offline experiences. Parents, educators, and caregivers are critical in guiding girls toward a balanced approach. Setting boundaries around screen time is one of the most effective ways to ensure healthy digital habits. Parents and caregivers can establish daily or weekly limits on screen use, encouraging girls to allocate time for outdoor play, reading, or hobbies. Introducing screen-free zones, such as during meals or before bedtime, helps reinforce the importance of disconnecting from devices and focusing on in-person interactions.

Not all screen time is equal. Helping girls differentiate between productive and passive screen use can enhance the quality of their online experiences. Educational apps, creative platforms, and tools that promote skill-building or learning can be prioritized over endless scrolling or gaming. Encouraging intentional use of technology ensures that screen time adds value rather than becoming a source of mindless distraction.

Creating opportunities for offline engagement is essential for striking a balance. Girls should be encouraged to explore activities that foster creativity, physical fitness, and social connection. Hobbies such as painting, playing a musical instrument, or participating in team sports provide fulfilling alternatives to screen use. Family outings and group activities can also strengthen relationships and create lasting memories away from digital devices.

Social media poses unique challenges that extend beyond screen time limits. Girls must be equipped with the tools to navigate these platforms responsibly and safeguard their mental health.

Teaching girls to critically evaluate the content they encounter online is a key skill in fostering resilience against social media's negative impacts. They can develop a more realistic perspective on what they see by helping them understand that many posts are edited, filtered, or staged. Discussions about the motives behind influencers and advertisers also promote skepticism and discourage unhealthy comparisons.

Girls should be educated about online safety practices, including setting strong passwords, understanding privacy settings, and recognizing phishing attempts. Encouraging them to think twice before sharing personal information or interacting with strangers online can help prevent potential risks. Building awareness about digital footprints ensures they understand the long-term implications of their online behavior.

Promoting kindness and empathy in digital communication is crucial for creating a positive online experience. Girls should be encouraged to think about the impact of their words and actions online, fostering a culture of respect and inclusivity. While cyberbullying and cyber abuse are addressed in another chapter, teaching proactive strategies such as blocking or reporting harmful content can empower girls to take control of their online environments.

Parents and caregivers often struggle to manage their children's screen time effectively. Providing them with tools and resources such as parental controls, monitoring apps, and guidelines for age-appropriate content can alleviate these challenges. Modeling balanced screen use is equally important; when adults demonstrate healthy habits, girls are likelier to emulate them.

Educational institutions and community organizations can support families in promoting balanced technology use. Schools can integrate lessons on digital citizenship, media literacy, and time management into their curricula. Community programs that encourage outdoor activities, group projects, and social interaction provide additional outlets for offline engagement.

Balancing online and offline life is essential to fostering mental and emotional well-being in girls. By establishing boundaries, encouraging mindful use of technology, and promoting meaningful offline activities, we can empower girls to navigate the digital world without compromising their personal growth. As they learn to balance the benefits of technology with the richness of offline experiences, girls are better equipped to lead healthy, fulfilling lives in an increasingly connected world.

Did you know?

- *Girls who regularly practice positive self-talk are less likely to develop body dissatisfaction and more likely to report higher confidence in school and friendships. Even simple daily affirmations can reshape how they see themselves.*
- *Research shows that teens who set daily screen time limits (such as no screens one hour before bed) report better sleep quality, higher self-esteem, and less anxiety compared to those who use devices without boundaries.*

A Few Words About Sex Education

At some point, every parent faces the inevitable question from their child: "How did I come into this world?" This seemingly innocent question often stirs unease as parents grapple with how much information to share and when. Early childhood curiosity, manifested in behaviors such as exploring their bodies, peeking under clothing, or comparing with peers, evolves into a deeper awareness as children grow older. First, crushes, dating, masturbation, and eventual sexual activity become a natural progression, leaving parents anxious about guiding their children through these milestones.

The approach to sex education varies widely and is influenced by cultural norms, family values, and individual beliefs. These perspectives often fall into three general categories:

- ❖ **Conservative Approaches**: In highly traditional families, discussions about sex are strictly avoided. Questions may be met with silence or even reprimands, leaving children to seek answers elsewhere.
- ❖ **Permissive Approaches**: In some families, nudity and openness about the body are normalized. Discussions about sex may occur freely, viewed as a natural part of life.
- ❖ **Misguided Practices**: Tragically, in rare cases, individuals misuse the concept of sex education for abusive purposes, such as framing inappropriate behaviors as "educational." These instances underline the importance of protecting children and establishing clear boundaries.

Sex education is deeply rooted in cultural and religious contexts. For example:

- In some societies, child marriages are normalized, with girls married off before reaching adolescence.
- Conversely, certain traditions discourage marriage altogether for specific children, expecting them to care for aging parents.
- Some African tribes practice marriage preparation schools, where young girls are sent to live with their future mothers-

in-law to learn the skills of homemaking, child-rearing, and marital duties.

Such practices underscore the diverse global perspectives on sexuality and the complexity of addressing sex education universally.

Sex education is not a one-size-fits-all process. It encompasses a blend of family, personal, and societal contributions:

1. **Parental Responsibility**: Some parents take a proactive approach, offering guidance and answering their children's questions about relationships, reproduction, and sexual health.
2. **Institutional Support**: Other families rely on schools to provide structured sex education programs.
3. **Independent Learning**: In some cases, children turn to books, the internet, or peers to fill the gaps in their knowledge.

Effective sex education hinges on creating an environment of open communication and trust. Parents and educators must approach this topic with honesty, sensitivity, and age-appropriate information. When done well, sex education empowers children to make informed and responsible decisions about their relationships and bodies.

Sex education is not a one-time conversation but a continuous process that evolves as children mature. The information shared should align with the child's cognitive and emotional development at every stage.

Children are naturally curious and may ask unexpected questions about sex at inconvenient moments, perhaps in public or during family gatherings. While these instances may feel uncomfortable, they present opportunities for honest, age-appropriate discussions. Parents should avoid dismissing or reprimanding their children, which could stifle curiosity and trust. For example, if a child asks why parents hug or kiss or even why certain noises are heard from their bedroom, they can answer calmly and respectfully without overexplaining.

For adolescent girls, discussions about sexuality are often intertwined with their relationship with their mothers. As girls experience changes such as menstruation, these conversations take on a more practical dimension. Unlike boys, whose initial interest in sex is often physical, girls are more likely to focus on the emotional aspects of relationships, such as love, intimacy, and affection.

Children should learn about the structure and function of reproductive organs. Girls, for example, must understand that menstruation signals the possibility of pregnancy. Topics should also include the differences between male and female anatomy, the changes during puberty, and the processes of conception and childbirth.

Children may experience physical sensations they don't fully understand as they mature. Educating them about bodily responses to touch, hugs, and kisses can prevent confusion or fear. For example:

- Girls may feel embarrassed when looking at their naked bodies in the mirror.
- Some may notice uterine contractions resembling an orgasm during dreams or specific phases of their cycle.

It's crucial to reassure children that these reactions are natural and part of growing up.

Every family has its views on relationships, shaped by religion, culture, and morality. While sharing these values with children is essential, they should not be imposed through force or fear.

Many parents hesitate to discuss their own experiences with unprotected sex or its consequences. However, these conversations are vital. Adolescents should understand:

- How to protect themselves against sexually transmitted infections (STIs).
- The availability and use of modern contraceptives.
- Emergency contraception options, particularly for girls.

Schools often address these topics, but parents play a crucial role in reinforcing this knowledge.

Sexual communication is a cornerstone of healthy relationships. Teaching adolescents to respectfully discuss their feelings, boundaries, and concerns lays the foundation for trust-based interactions with future partners. This skill also strengthens parent-child relationships, ensuring open dialogue on sensitive topics.

Girls are disproportionately affected by sexual violence. Education must focus on:

1. **How to identify and avoid dangerous situations.**
2. **How to respond effectively if violence occurs.**

Programs offering self-defense training can empower adolescents to protect themselves physically and emotionally.

Sex education should extend beyond the physical to include lessons on building mutual respect, understanding, and trust. Parents serve as role models in this regard. Children observe how their parents interact and often emulate these behaviors in their relationships.

In today's digital age, parents and educators have access to a wealth of books, videos, and online platforms dedicated to sex education. While these resources are valuable, they should complement, not replace, direct conversations between parents and children. Personal interaction remains the cornerstone of adequate sex education.

By fostering open, honest, and supportive discussions, parents and educators can equip children with the tools they need to navigate their sexual development responsibly and confidently.

Did You Know?

- *Young children's questions about their bodies and reproduction are natural expressions of curiosity, not a sign of premature sexualization. Addressing these questions calmly lays the groundwork for open communication later in life.*
- *Studies show that adolescents who receive comprehensive sex education are more likely to delay sexual activity and use protection when they do become sexually active, reducing risks of STIs and unplanned pregnancies.*

Gender Transition and Parental Perspectives

Every parent envisions a future for their child - a "perfect adult" they hope to see one day: **healthy, educated, prosperous, and virtuous**. This vision often reflects the parents' ideals and aspirations rather than the child's evolving sense of self. Parents accept changes in their child's dreams about careers or hobbies, but one aspect of this vision, gender identity, and sexual orientation, is often presumed to align with traditional norms.

When children express a nontraditional sexual orientation or gender identity, this can be a profoundly disorienting moment for parents. Discovering that a child identifies as homosexual, bisexual, or transgender may evoke feelings of confusion, shame, anger, or betrayal. In some cases, this leads to rejection, punishment, and attempts to suppress or alter the child's identity, causing profound emotional harm.

Today, the acronym **LGBT** (Lesbian, Gay, Bisexual, Transgender) represents individuals with nontraditional sexual orientations and gender identities. Though LGBT individuals constitute a minority of the global population, more people are openly identifying with these groups. Social awareness has grown, but stigmatization and misunderstanding persist.

Parents may react in two main ways when a child exhibits nontraditional sexual behavior or questions their gender identity:

- ❖ **Protest or Rebellion**
    - For some adolescents, nontraditional behavior arises as **defiance** against strict parenting.
    - When parents enforce rigid rules about interactions with peers—particularly of the opposite sex—children may rebel, exploring what has been forbidden.
    - This rebellion may manifest as a phase of experimentation rather than a reflection of true gender identity or sexual orientation.
- ❖ **Authentic Nontraditional Identity**

- For others, nontraditional behavior is an **authentic expression** of their identity.
- These children are not rebelling but seeking acknowledgment and acceptance of their genuine identity.

In both cases, parental reactions are critical in shaping the child's self-esteem, emotional health, and ability to navigate their world.

Children who identify as LGBT often face external challenges such as bullying, discrimination, and societal rejection. The parent-child relationship becomes a lifeline during this time. Supportive parents can mitigate the emotional harm caused by external negativity, while rejection can exacerbate feelings of isolation, depression, and anxiety.

By fostering open communication, showing empathy, and demonstrating unconditional love, parents can create a safe space for their children to thrive emotionally and socially, regardless of their gender identity or sexual orientation.

Twenty years ago, discussions about gender transition were rare and often clouded by negativity and condemnation. Today, these conversations are more frequent, though societal attitudes remain divided. In many countries, expressing transgender identity or pursuing transition still results in legal, professional, and social repercussions. In contrast, many developed nations now address the topic openly, reducing stigma and fostering inclusion.

Statistics from the United States indicate that approximately 1 in 137 adolescents aged 13-17 identifies as transgender. However, a much smaller percentage pursue medical or surgical interventions for gender transition.

Transgender adolescents often face unique challenges, including:

- Mental health struggles, such as depression and anxiety.
- Higher suicide rates compared to their peers.
- Risk of homelessness, often resulting from family rejection.
- Difficulties accessing medical care for hormonal therapy or gender-affirming procedures can be expensive and complex.

Children are not born with a clear understanding of gender identity—these concepts are taught through interactions with family, peers, and society. From the moment of birth, gender is assigned based on the external genitalia, and societal norms dictate expectations for boys and girls:

- Girls are given pink clothing, dolls, and accessories emphasizing femininity.
- Boys are dressed in blue and encouraged to engage in masculine behaviors.

While these norms may seem straightforward, a child's sense of self is far more complex. Gender identity is influenced by biological, psychological, and social factors, and science is still uncovering its intricacies.

For parents, understanding and supporting a transgender child requires empathy and education.

1. **Open Communication**
    - Encourage honest, judgment-free discussions about your child's feelings and experiences.
2. **Respect Name and Pronoun Preferences**
    - Acknowledging your child's chosen name and pronouns validates their identity and fosters trust.
3. **Explore Transition Options Together**
    - Gender transition can include social changes (e.g., name, clothing) and medical interventions (e.g., hormonal therapy or surgery).
    - Discussing these options can help your child feel supported, even if the family cannot immediately pursue medical treatments.
4. **Advocate Against Transphobia**
    - Defend your child against transphobic attitudes or actions, whether from extended family, peers, or institutions.
5. **Educate Yourself**
    - Learn about transgender issues to better understand your child's journey.

Medical professionals increasingly advocate for early support for gender transitions. Research indicates that transitioning before puberty simplifies the process and minimizes psychological harm. Hormonal therapies are most effective when started early, though they require lifelong medical monitoring.

While these treatments can be costly and complex, their benefits often outweigh the risks, particularly for adolescents experiencing severe gender dysphoria.

For many parents, accepting a transgender child can feel overwhelming or even painful. However, it is crucial to understand that neither the parents nor the child is at fault. Rather than viewing gender identity as a problem to be fixed, parents should embrace their child's unique journey with love and understanding.

By creating a home environment that prioritizes **acceptance, support, and education**, families can empower their transgender children to thrive despite societal challenges.

Did You Know?

- *Transgender Adolescents Face Higher Mental Health Risks: Studies show that transgender youth are significantly more likely to experience depression, anxiety, and suicidal thoughts, mainly due to societal rejection and lack of support. Family acceptance can dramatically reduce these risks.*
- *Early Support for Gender Identity Reduces Dysphoria: Providing affirming care, such as using a child's chosen name and pronouns, can improve mental health outcomes and help transgender youth navigate their identity with confidence.*

Girls' Safety and Sexual Harassment

Despite significant advancements in legislation, the expansion of law enforcement systems, the introduction of sex education in schools, and the availability of various resources, sexual violence remains a deeply rooted societal issue. It is a problem that transcends borders, cultures, and social classes, leaving a trail of emotional, psychological, and physical harm in its wake. The trauma associated with sexual violence often reverberates far beyond the immediate event, affecting victims' self-esteem, mental health, relationships, and ability to feel safe in the world.

Sexual violence encompasses a spectrum of harmful behaviors, from verbal harassment and coercion to physical assault. At its core, these acts are rooted in an abuse of power and a disregard for consent, reducing the victim to an object of dominance rather than an autonomous individual. To effectively combat sexual violence, society must develop a deeper understanding of its manifestations and take proactive steps to prevent and address these acts.

Violence, in its broadest sense, is the use of physical, verbal, or psychological force to impose one's will, causing harm to another. It manifests in various forms: physical, verbal, emotional, sexual, financial, and even religious violence. Abuse, by contrast, refers to the exploitation or misuse of trust, relationships, or circumstances for selfish or harmful purposes. Both are often intertwined, creating a cycle of harm that is difficult to break.

Among these, sexual violence is particularly devastating. It represents a profound violation of personal boundaries, leaving victims to grapple with a mix of emotions — shame, fear, anger, and betrayal. Sexual harassment, as a subset of sexual violence, includes behaviors intended to intimidate, demean, or coerce a person. Examples range from inappropriate jokes and verbal comments to unwelcome physical contact and overt acts of molestation. In some jurisdictions, even prolonged or "lingering" stares are recognized as harassment, highlighting the evolving understanding of consent and personal boundaries.

The digital era has introduced new dimensions to sexual violence. While technology offers countless benefits, it has also become a tool for predators who exploit its anonymity and reach. Online harassment is an escalating concern, with alarming statistics underscoring its prevalence:

- Approximately 1 in 7 young people report receiving sexual propositions online.
- Nearly 10% of adolescents have been sent explicit images or messages without their consent.
- 76% of sexual violence cases involving adolescents originate from interactions in online chats.
- In nearly 50% of these cases, perpetrators entice victims with promises of gifts or money.
- Up to 15% of girls aged 12-17 have received sexually explicit content on their mobile devices.

One particularly concerning trend is sexting, the exchange of sexually explicit messages or images. Over 25% of teenagers engage in sexting, often underestimating its potential consequences. These exchanges can lead to blackmail, public humiliation, or coercion into further acts of exploitation. The psychological impact on victims can be as severe as that of in-person abuse, with many experiencing anxiety, depression, and feelings of isolation.

A significant danger of online communication lies in the false sense of security it provides. Children and adolescents often develop trust in virtual relationships, unaware of the risks. Predators exploit this vulnerability, using grooming tactics to manipulate their victims over time. These interactions can escalate from seemingly harmless conversations to severe exploitation, further emphasizing the importance of parental vigilance and digital literacy.

Parents must educate their children about the risks of online interactions and encourage open communication. Establishing a safe space for discussing uncomfortable or suspicious encounters is crucial in mitigating potential harm.

It is an uncomfortable truth that most perpetrators of sexual violence are not strangers but individuals known to the victim. Family members, neighbors, friends, and acquaintances often exploit their proximity and the trust placed in them. Recognizing the signs of abuse is essential in protecting children and ensuring timely intervention.

Young children may not understand that inappropriate touching or behavior is wrong. Perpetrators often bribe or intimidate them into silence, using candy, toys, money, or threats. Parents should watch for behavioral changes or unusual actions during play, such as:

- Mimicking explicit actions, like undressing dolls or reenacting adult gestures.
- Repeating words or phrases that seem out of context for their age.

In cases of suspicion, consulting a child psychologist can help clarify the situation and guide appropriate action.

Adolescents respond to trauma differently. Their reactions might include withdrawal, irritability, mood swings, or a sudden loss of interest in activities they once enjoyed. These behaviors are often dismissed as typical teenage moodiness, making it essential for parents to approach such changes with sensitivity and awareness.

How Parents Should Respond

When a child discloses sexual harassment or abuse, a parent's response can profoundly influence their recovery process. Reacting with support and care is crucial in helping the child feel safe and understood. Key steps include:

1. Listen Without Interruption: Allow the child to share their story fully without interjecting or questioning excessively.

2. Stay Calm: Suppress visible anger or panic, as these reactions may discourage the child from continuing to open up.
3. Believe the Child: Trust their account, even if the details seem implausible or shocking.
4. Reassure Them: Emphasize that they are not at fault and did nothing to deserve what happened.
5. Focus on Support: Offer emotional and psychological support without dwelling excessively on their victimhood.
6. Discuss Next Steps: Collaborate with the child to determine how best to proceed, whether through therapy, medical care, or legal action.
7. Address Physical Health: Seek medical evaluation to address potential injuries or exposure to sexually transmitted infections.
8. Be Present: Spend quality time with the child to rebuild their sense of safety and trust.
9. Express Unconditional Love: Reinforce that they are valued and supported, no matter what.

Prevention is a shared responsibility that requires coordinated efforts from parents, schools, communities, and governments. Creating a culture of safety and respect involves education, empowerment, and vigilance.

Schools are pivotal in teaching children about consent, boundaries, and reporting inappropriate behavior. These programs should also address the responsibilities of boys and young men, fostering a culture of respect and accountability.

Self-defense classes and assertiveness training can equip girls with the skills and confidence to protect themselves. Teaching them to recognize and respond to potentially dangerous situations is a vital aspect of empowerment.

Governments must continue to refine and enforce laws that protect victims and prosecute offenders. Equally important is training law enforcement officers to handle cases with sensitivity and respect.

Parents should foster an environment where children feel comfortable discussing sensitive topics. Open dialogue can demystify issues surrounding consent and boundaries, making children more likely to report concerns.

It is crucial to teach children how to navigate online spaces safely. This includes recognizing red flags, understanding privacy settings, and knowing how to report harassment or abuse.

Addressing sexual violence is a complex challenge that requires vigilance, education, and collaboration. Parents, educators, and communities can create a safer environment for girls and young women by fostering open dialogue, promoting awareness, and ensuring access to support systems. Recognizing the evolving dynamics of real-life and digital threats is essential in protecting the next generation and empowering them to navigate their environments confidently and resiliently.

Did You Know?

- *Most Sexual Violence Cases Involve Acquaintances: Contrary to common assumptions, over 80% of sexual violence incidents are perpetrated by someone the victim knows, such as a family member, friend, or neighbor.*
- *Online harassment Affects a Significant Number of Adolescents: Nearly 25% of teenagers have engaged in sexting or been victims of unsolicited explicit content online, highlighting the growing need for digital literacy and parental guidance.*

Cyberviolence and Cyberbullying: The Invisible Threat

Many people approach terms like cyberviolence and cyberbullying with indifference, often unaware of their devastating implications. It wasn't until the widespread tragedy of the online game "Blue Whale" emerged that society began to confront the lurking dangers of cyberspace. This seemingly innocuous "game" entrapped tens of thousands of children in a deadly cycle of manipulation, culminating in self-harm and, tragically, suicide for some.

The case revealed a startling truth: the internet, often perceived as a harmless tool for communication and entertainment, can harbor profound threats. More disturbingly, it highlighted a glaring gap: most parents and guardians were woefully unprepared to recognize or combat these dangers. While rich with opportunity, the digital landscape has proven to be an equally fertile ground for harm.

At its core, **cyber violence** involves the use of electronic communication tools — social media, messaging apps, email, and online forums — to harm, intimidate, or manipulate individuals. **Cyberbullying**, a subset of cyberviolence, refers specifically to harassment or bullying conducted in the digital realm.

Unlike traditional bullying, cyberviolence operates without boundaries. It can strike at any time, in any place, leaving victims with little refuge. The internet's capacity for instant information exchange magnifies its impact, turning private matters into public spectacles in mere moments.

Characteristics of Cyberviolence:

1. **Relentless Nature:** Unlike face-to-face bullying, cyberviolence is persistent. Victims can receive harmful messages or threats at all hours, invading even the sanctity of their homes.
2. **Anonymity:** The digital world allows perpetrators to hide behind screens, making it easier to escape accountability while emboldening their actions.

3. **Global Reach:** In seconds, a single post, rumor, or image can spread across the globe, amplifying the victim's humiliation and despair.

These attributes make cyberviolence uniquely damaging, creating an environment where psychological harm often eclipses the physical.

The truth is that **anyone** can fall prey to cyber violence. While adults are not immune, children and adolescents are disproportionately affected. Their heavy reliance on digital communication for socialization and validation renders them particularly vulnerable. Teenagers often forge deep emotional connections online, trusting peers or even strangers with personal details.

Among the most vulnerable groups are:

❖ Social Media Enthusiasts: Teens who actively share their lives online often expose themselves to risks, from ridicule to exploitation.

❖ Infrequent Users: Even those rarely engage online can fall victim to hacking, phishing, or blackmail.

Perpetrators precisely exploit these vulnerabilities, often manipulating victims into compliance or silence.

The actual scope of cyberviolence is staggering. While high-profile cases of teen suicides due to online harassment capture public attention, they are merely the tip of the iceberg. The harm extends far beyond these tragedies, leaving countless others emotionally scarred, socially isolated, and struggling with mental health issues.

Victims often face:

- Psychological Trauma: Depression, anxiety, and low self-esteem are common outcomes of persistent cyberbullying.
- Social Withdrawal: Many victims retreat from their social circles out of fear or shame, further exacerbating their isolation.
- Academic and Professional Setbacks**:** The mental toll of cyberviolence often interferes with school or work performance, affecting long-term prospects.

Society's challenge lies in addressing these issues proactively rather than reacting only after a crisis unfolds.

The devastating impact of cyberviolence is most evident in the stories of its victims. In 2003, Ryan Halligan, a 13-year-old boy, took his life after enduring relentless online bullying, including malicious rumors about his sexuality. Three years later, Megan Meier, also 13, became a victim of cyberbullying on MySpace, leading to her suicide.

One of the most harrowing cases came in 2010 with the death of Tyler Clementi, an 18-year-old college student. After discovering a video of him kissing another boy had been shared on Twitter without his consent, Tyler ended his life. These stories, though heartbreaking, have galvanized efforts to combat cyber violence, inspiring legislative action and advocacy campaigns.

Statistics reveal the grim reality of cyberviolence:

- Annually, 4,400 young people in the United States die by suicide, with over 100,000 attempts recorded. Among these, 7% are directly linked to cyberbullying.
- Adolescents aged 12–18 are the most frequent targets, with girls particularly susceptible to harassment involving body shaming or intimate image exploitation.
- 76% of cyberviolence cases begin with interactions in online chat rooms, often escalating into real-life threats or exploitation.

Cyberviolence can manifest in various forms, each uniquely harmful:

- **Spreading Rumors or False Information:** Publicly tarnishing someone's reputation through lies or half-truths.
- **Unauthorized Sharing:** Posting private photos or videos without consent, often to humiliate or blackmail.
- **Hacking and Impersonation:** Gaining unauthorized access to personal accounts to manipulate or harm the victim.
- **Public Shaming:** Using blogs, forums, or social media to ridicule or degrade individuals.

Perhaps most troubling is the passive role many play in perpetuating cyber violence. By sharing, liking, or observing harmful content, bystanders can unintentionally validate and amplify the abuse.

For parents and educators, recognizing and addressing cyberviolence is essential. While anger or punitive measures might feel instinctive, they are rarely effective. Instead, fostering trust and open communication with children is crucial.

Steps to take include:

- **Listening Without Judgment:** Allow the child to share their experience openly, without fear of reprimand.
- **Documenting Evidence:** Encourage them to save harmful messages, screenshots, or emails as evidence for reporting.
- **Seeking Help:** Report incidents to the support teams of social media platforms or law enforcement when necessary.
- **Providing Emotional Support:** Reassure the child that they are not alone and that help is available.

Preventing cyberviolence requires a holistic approach:

1. **Digital Literacy Education:** Teach children about safe online practices, such as protecting passwords and avoiding sharing personal information.
2. **Parental Engagement:** Stay informed about your child's online activities, maintaining a supportive presence without being intrusive.
3. **Community Collaboration:** Schools, community groups, and governments must work together to raise awareness and establish robust support systems.

Cyberviolence is not an isolated problem; it reflects broader societal challenges in adapting to the digital age. We can create a safer online environment by fostering empathy, promoting education, and providing accessible resources. It's a shared responsibility that demands vigilance, compassion, and action.

Let us not wait for the next tragedy to address the silent epidemic of cyber violence. Together, we can ensure the digital world becomes a space of connection and growth, not harm and despair.

Did You Know?

- *Cyberbullying Can Be Deadly: Annually, 7% of youth suicides in the United States are linked directly to cyberbullying, highlighting the critical need for awareness and intervention.*
- *Girls Are at Higher Risk: Adolescent girls are particularly vulnerable to cyber violence, with body shaming and intimate image exploitation being the most common forms of harassment they face.*

Environmental and Lifestyle Factors

A girl's health is intricately influenced by the environment she grows up in and the lifestyle choices she adopts. Though often overlooked, these factors play a critical role in shaping her physical, emotional, and cognitive development. From the air she breathes and the food she eats to her exposure to societal norms and daily habits, the interplay of environmental and lifestyle elements can have immediate and long-term impacts on her well-being.

The environment encompasses a wide range of physical and social determinants. Air and water quality, exposure to toxins, access to safe recreational spaces, and socioeconomic conditions are all external factors that can significantly affect a girl's health. For instance, prolonged exposure to polluted air is linked to respiratory issues and reduced cognitive function, while living in neighborhoods with limited green spaces can contribute to a sedentary lifestyle and mental health challenges.

On the other hand, lifestyle choices are shaped by family practices, cultural influences, and individual preferences. Nutrition, physical activity, sleep patterns, and screen time are pivotal in determining a girl's health. Poor dietary habits and insufficient physical activity can lead to obesity and associated chronic conditions, such as diabetes and cardiovascular issues. Similarly, irregular sleep patterns and excessive screen time are increasingly related to mental health challenges, including anxiety and depression.

Social environments and cultural norms further complicate these dynamics. Girls often face unique pressures related to body image, academic expectations, and social conformity, which can influence their choices and behaviors. Additionally, socioeconomic disparities can create barriers to accessing healthy food, safe living conditions, and quality healthcare, disproportionately affecting vulnerable populations.

This chapter delves into the myriad environmental and lifestyle factors that shape a girl's health, offering insights into their complex interactions. By understanding these influences, we can identify opportunities to create supportive environments and encourage positive lifestyle choices that promote lifelong health and resilience. Through targeted interventions and informed decision-making, we can empower girls to thrive in a world where their well-being is prioritized and nurtured.

Impact of Environmental Toxins

Environmental toxins represent one of the most concerning threats to girls' health, particularly during critical periods of development. Among these toxins, endocrine-disrupting chemicals (EDCs) stand out for their ability to interfere with the hormonal systems that regulate growth, metabolism, and reproduction. EDCs are pervasive in the modern environment and found in everyday products such as plastics, personal care items, pesticides, and industrial chemicals. Their widespread presence and potential for long-term health effects make them a significant focus of concern for children, especially girls.

EDCs are synthetic or naturally occurring compounds that mimic, block, or alter the body's hormonal signaling. Hormones are critical regulators of physiological processes, and even minor disruptions can profoundly affect a developing child. For girls whose hormonal systems are particularly sensitive during infancy, puberty, and adolescence, exposure to EDCs can lead to a range of adverse outcomes.

Common EDCs include:

- **Bisphenol A (BPA):** Found in plastics and food packaging, BPA is known to mimic estrogen, a key hormone in female development.
- **Phthalates:** Used in cosmetics, fragrances, and flexible plastics, these compounds can interfere with reproductive hormone activity.
- **Polychlorinated biphenyls (PCBs) and Dioxins:** Persistent environmental pollutants that accumulate in the food chain, affecting immune and reproductive health.

- **Pesticides:** Chemicals such as atrazine and organophosphates disrupt endocrine function and are linked to developmental disorders.

Exposure to EDCs during sensitive developmental windows can have both immediate and long-term effects on girls' health. Key areas of concern include:

❖ **Reproductive Health:**

EDCs such as BPA and phthalates have been associated with the early onset of puberty in girls, a condition linked to increased risks of breast cancer, obesity, and mental health challenges later in life. Disruption of estrogen and progesterone pathways can result in menstrual irregularities and reduced fertility in adulthood.

❖ **Neurodevelopmental Effects:**

Studies suggest that prenatal and early-life exposure to EDCs may impair cognitive function and increase the risk of neurodevelopmental disorders such as ADHD and learning disabilities. Hormonal disruptions during brain development can affect mood regulation and stress responses, contributing to anxiety and depression in adolescence.

❖ **Obesity and Metabolic Disorders:**

Some EDCs, referred to as "obesogens," interfere with metabolic processes, increasing the likelihood of weight gain and related conditions such as diabetes and cardiovascular disease.

❖ **Immune System Dysregulation:**

Persistent organic pollutants like PCBs and dioxins can weaken immune responses, making girls more susceptible to infections and autoimmune conditions.

Understanding the sources of EDC exposure is crucial for developing effective prevention strategies. Common exposure pathways include:

- **Diet:** EDCs can enter the body through contaminated food and water. Pesticides on produce and chemicals leaching from plastic containers are significant contributors.
- **Household Products:** Cleaning agents, cosmetics, and personal care items often contain phthalates and other endocrine disruptors.

- **Environmental Contamination:** Proximity to industrial sites, agricultural areas, or polluted water sources increases the likelihood of EDC exposure.

Understanding the sources of EDC exposure is crucial for developing effective prevention strategies. Common exposure pathways include:

- To reduce pesticide and chemical intake, encourage the consumption of organic produce and minimally processed foods. Avoid heating food in plastic containers to minimize BPA exposure.
- Opt for cosmetics and personal care items labeled "phthalate-free" or "paraben-free." Look for non-toxic household cleaning alternatives.
- Support regulations that limit harmful chemicals in consumer products and promote clean-up efforts in contaminated areas.
- Raise awareness about EDCs and their health impacts to empower families to make informed choices and advocate for safer environments.

The pervasive presence of endocrine-disrupting chemicals in the environment poses significant risks to girls' health, particularly during critical periods of growth and development. By understanding the sources and impacts of EDC exposure, we can take proactive steps to minimize risks and promote healthier outcomes. Protecting girls from these invisible yet harmful toxins is not only a matter of individual action but also requires collective advocacy for systemic change. Through education, prevention, and policy reform, we can safeguard the health and future of the next generation.

Sleep Patterns in Adolescence

Adolescence is a transformative period marked by rapid physical, emotional, and cognitive development. During this stage, sleep becomes essential to overall health, playing a critical role in memory consolidation, emotional regulation, and physical growth. However, the sleep patterns of adolescents, particularly girls, are often disrupted by a combination of biological changes and societal demands, leading to a concerning trend of sleep deprivation.

Adequate sleep is vital for maintaining optimal health and well-being during adolescence. Research indicates that teenagers require 8 to 10 hours of sleep per night to support their developmental needs. Sufficient sleep is linked to improved academic performance, better mood stability, and enhanced physical health for girls. Sleep also plays a critical role in regulating hormones influencing appetite, growth, and reproductive health.

Sleep deprivation, on the other hand, has far-reaching consequences. Chronic sleep can impair cognitive function, reduce attention span, and negatively affect decision-making skills. Emotionally, insufficient sleep is associated with increased levels of stress, anxiety, and depression, issues that are particularly prevalent among adolescent girls due to societal pressures and hormonal fluctuations.

Biological changes during adolescence alter the circadian rhythm, the internal clock that regulates sleep-wake cycles. During puberty, the release of melatonin, a hormone that promotes sleep, is delayed, causing a natural shift in the timing of sleepiness. This phenomenon, known as a "sleep phase delay," makes it difficult for teenagers to fall asleep early and wake up in time for school or other morning commitments.

For adolescent girls, this shift is compounded by additional factors such as academic responsibilities, extracurricular activities, and social engagements. Many girls also experience heightened sensitivity to stress and anxiety, which can further delay the onset of sleep and contribute to restless nights. The increased use of electronic devices before bedtime exacerbates the problem, as blue light exposure suppresses melatonin production and disrupts the circadian rhythm.

Given the critical importance of sleep, addressing the factors that disrupt healthy sleep patterns in adolescent girls is essential.

Promoting good sleep hygiene and creating supportive environments can mitigate the adverse effects of sleep deprivation.

1. **Establishing Consistent Sleep Schedules:** Encouraging girls to go to bed and wake up at the same time every day, even on weekends, helps regulate the circadian rhythm and improves sleep quality.
2. **Limiting Screen Time Before Bed:** Reducing exposure to electronic devices at least one hour before bedtime minimizes blue light interference with melatonin production. Introducing relaxing pre-sleep routines, such as reading or practicing mindfulness, can aid in winding down.
3. **Creating a Sleep-Friendly Environment:** Ensuring the bedroom is quiet, dark, and comfortable promotes restful sleep. Blackout curtains, white noise machines, and comfy bedding can enhance the sleeping environment.
4. **Managing Stress and Anxiety:** Teaching stress management techniques, such as deep breathing exercises or journaling, can help girls relax and prepare for sleep. Addressing academic pressures and promoting open communication about emotional challenges are also key.
5. **Balancing Responsibilities:** Encouraging a balanced approach to school, extracurriculars, and social activities can prevent overcommitment and reduce the likelihood of sleep deprivation.

Sleep is a cornerstone of health during adolescence, yet many girls face significant challenges in achieving adequate rest. By understanding the biological and environmental factors that affect sleep patterns, we can implement strategies to promote better sleep hygiene and support their overall well-being. Prioritizing sleep enhances academic and emotional outcomes and lays the foundation for a lifetime of healthy habits.

Did you know?

- *Everyday items like plastic bottles, cosmetics, and even some cleaning products can contain chemicals that mimic hormones, affecting puberty and long-term health in girls.*

Transition to Adulthood (18-21 Years)

The transition to adulthood marks a pivotal stage in a girl's life, encompassing significant physical, emotional, and social changes. Between 18 and 21, girls often experience a shift in responsibilities, independence, and identity formation. This period is characterized by milestones such as higher education, career exploration, and the development of deeper interpersonal relationships. At the same time, it presents unique challenges as girls navigate the complexities of adulthood while managing their health and well-being.

During this transitional phase, maintaining a healthy lifestyle becomes increasingly evident. The habits and choices established during these years often set the foundation for long-term health outcomes. Nutritional needs evolve, stress levels may rise due to academic and career pressures, and social environments usually expand to include diverse influences. Understanding how to balance these demands with self-care is essential for fostering resilience and overall well-being for young women.

The goal is to empower girls with the tools they need to thrive during this transformative time, from managing stress and building supportive networks to making informed decisions about nutrition and exercise.

Health Screenings for Young Women

Health screenings are a cornerstone of preventative care, offering young women a proactive approach to maintaining their well-being during adulthood. Between 18 and 21, regular medical checkups become increasingly important as young women take ownership of their health. Among these, gynecological exams and screenings for sexually transmitted infections (STIs) play a pivotal role in detecting potential issues early and ensuring long-term health. While the specifics of sexually transmitted diseases (STDs) are discussed in a separate chapter, this section focuses on the importance of regular screenings and the role they play in fostering overall well-being.

Gynecological exams are essential to women's health care, particularly as young women transition into adulthood. These exams serve multiple purposes, including:

- **Monitoring Reproductive Health:** Routine pelvic exams allow healthcare providers to assess the health of the reproductive organs and identify any abnormalities, such as ovarian cysts or uterine fibroids, that may require further investigation.
- **Cervical Cancer Screening:** Pap smears, recommended at age 21, are critical in detecting precancerous changes in the cervix caused by human papillomavirus (HPV) infections. Early detection significantly reduces the risk of cervical cancer.
- **Addressing Menstrual and Hormonal Concerns:** Gynecological visits provide an opportunity to discuss irregular periods, hormonal imbalances, or symptoms of conditions like polycystic ovary syndrome (PCOS), which can impact overall health and fertility.
- **Contraception and Family Planning:** For sexually active young women, gynecological exams offer a safe space to discuss contraceptive options and receive guidance on family planning, ensuring that choices align with individual needs and goals.

Regular gynecological exams also promote self-awareness and empowerment, encouraging young women to take an active role in their health. Establishing a relationship with a trusted healthcare provider fosters open communication and ensures that any concerns are addressed promptly.

Screening for sexually transmitted infections is another critical aspect of health care for young women. Regular STI screenings help identify infections early, often before symptoms appear, reducing the risk of complications and transmission to others. Standard STI screenings include tests for chlamydia, gonorrhea, and syphilis, as well as blood tests for HIV and hepatitis

B and C. Early detection allows for timely treatment, minimizing long-term health impacts such as infertility or chronic pain.

In addition to STI screenings, this stage of life is an ideal time to address other health conditions that may arise. Young women should be screened for:

- **Mental Health Concerns:** Depression, anxiety, and stress are prevalent among young adults, making mental health screenings an essential part of regular checkups.
- **Nutritional Deficiencies:** Tests for iron levels and other nutrients ensure that dietary habits support overall health.
- **Blood Pressure and Cholesterol Levels:** Monitoring these markers helps identify early signs of cardiovascular risk factors, enabling preventative measures.

The transition to adulthood is a time of significant growth and change, and regular health screenings provide young women with the tools to navigate this period confidently. By prioritizing gynecological exams and STI screenings, young women can address potential health concerns proactively and establish habits that support their well-being. Additionally, these screenings serve as a gateway to broader discussions about health, empowering young women to make informed decisions and advocate for themselves in healthcare settings.

Regular checkups safeguard physical health and foster independence and self-awareness. By emphasizing the importance of preventive care, we can help young women build a foundation for lifelong health, ensuring they are equipped to thrive in every aspect of their lives.

Managing Stress and Mental Health in College or Work Life

The transition to college or a demanding work environment often marks a significant shift in a young woman's life, presenting opportunities and challenges. For girls and young women, these transitions can be compounded by societal expectations, gender-specific stressors, and unique health concerns. Balancing academic, professional, and personal responsibilities often requires intentional effort to maintain mental and physical well-being.

Stress can manifest differently in young women than men, often influenced by hormonal changes and societal pressures. For example, girls may experience heightened stress during adolescence or young adulthood due to academic expectations, body image concerns, or navigating relationships. Chronic stress can affect menstrual health, sleep patterns, and emotional well-being, potentially leading to long-term health issues if not addressed.

Mental health challenges such as anxiety and depression are prevalent among young women in high-pressure environments. Recognizing the early signs, such as persistent fatigue, changes in eating habits, or withdrawal from social activities, is essential for timely intervention.

Strategies for Managing Stress

1. **Holistic Health Practices:** Encourage young women to adopt a holistic approach to health, integrating balanced nutrition, regular exercise, and mindfulness practices like yoga or meditation.
2. **Open Conversations:** Girls often benefit from having trusted mentors or counselors to discuss their challenges. Creating safe spaces for open dialogue about stress, self-esteem, and personal goals is invaluable.
3. **Menstrual Health Awareness:** Understanding how stress impacts the menstrual cycle, and hormonal balance can help girls manage symptoms effectively. Resources like period tracking apps and consultations with healthcare professionals can provide insights.
4. **Community and Peer Support:** Building connections with supportive peers or participating in women-centric groups can foster a sense of belonging and resilience.

5. **Professional Resources:** Accessing mental health services, including therapy or counseling, is essential for addressing severe stress or emotional challenges. Universities and workplaces often offer tailored resources for young women.

By prioritizing these strategies, girls and young women can build resilience, navigate the complexities of academic and professional life, and maintain their health and well-being.

Financial literacy is vital for girls and young women, empowering them to make informed decisions about their health and future. In some countries, medical services are free, alleviating financial burdens for individuals. However, understanding health insurance and medical costs in many regions remains crucial.

Health insurance is a key component of managing medical costs, yet many young women lack familiarity with its intricacies. Key terms to understand include:

- Premiums: The monthly payment required to maintain insurance coverage.
- Deductibles: The amount paid out-of-pocket before insurance starts covering medical costs.
- Co-pays and Co-insurance: The shared cost of medical services after meeting the deductible.
- Out-of-Pocket Maximums: The maximum an individual will pay in a year, after which insurance covers all eligible expenses.

For young women, selecting a plan should account for specific needs, such as coverage for gynecological care, contraceptives, or maternity services. Researching plans with preventive care benefits is especially valuable.

Financial education tailored to young women should include lessons on budgeting for healthcare, understanding prescription costs, and utilizing tools like Health Savings Accounts (HSAs). Fostering discussions about financial independence and planning for long-term health needs encourages self-sufficiency.
By equipping girls with financial literacy, they can better navigate the healthcare system, ensuring their physical and mental health

needs are met without undue financial burden. This foundational skill empowers them to prioritize well-being, paving the way for a healthier and more secure future.

Did you know?

- *The first Pap smear is recommended at age 21—even if a young woman isn't sexually active. Early screening can detect precancerous changes caused by HPV, dramatically lowering the risk of cervical cancer.*
- *Nearly 1 in 3 college-aged women report experiencing anxiety or depression, with stress often linked to academic pressures, financial concerns, and body image. Early recognition and support can make a lasting difference in mental health.*

Chronic Conditions and Disabilities

Managing chronic conditions and ensuring adequate healthcare for girls with disabilities are critical aspects of promoting equitable and inclusive health practices. Girls and young women often face unique challenges in accessing care, understanding their conditions, and navigating healthcare systems, which can impact their overall quality of life.

Chronic conditions such as diabetes, asthma, and autoimmune disorders require ongoing care and management. For girls and young women, managing these conditions often intersects with their educational, social, and emotional development, making tailored support essential.

❖ ***Diabetes Management***

- Educating girls about the nature of diabetes, including the importance of blood sugar monitoring and the role of insulin, is vital. Early education ensures that young women can manage their condition with confidence.
- Proper nutrition is a cornerstone of diabetes management. Girls benefit from learning how to make healthy food choices, especially during growth phases when dietary needs change. Schools and families can play a key role in promoting balanced meals.
- Managing a chronic condition like diabetes can be emotionally taxing. Support groups, counseling, or school-based programs can help girls cope with feelings of isolation or anxiety related to their condition.

❖ ***Asthma Management***

- Ensuring girls have access to prescribed inhalers and preventive medications is critical for effectively managing asthma symptoms.
- Educating girls about common asthma triggers such as allergens, pollution, or stress can empower them to minimize risks and take control of their health.

- Girls with asthma should be encouraged to participate in physical activities, with adjustments as needed. Sports programs can promote inclusion by accommodating specific health needs.

Regular visits to healthcare providers are essential for monitoring conditions and making necessary adjustments to treatment plans. Connecting girls with peers facing similar challenges fosters a sense of community and reduces feelings of isolation. Engaged and informed caregivers support girls' adherence to treatment and promote healthy habits.

Girls with disabilities face unique health challenges and barriers that require tailored approaches to ensure comprehensive care. These barriers may include physical access issues, communication difficulties, and a lack of understanding from healthcare providers.

Regular health checkups should include screenings for common conditions and attention to specific risks associated with certain disabilities. For instance, girls with mobility impairments may have higher risks of developing osteoporosis or pressure sores. Girls with disabilities may experience increased risks of depression and anxiety due to societal stigma or isolation. Providing access to counseling or support groups helps address these challenges. They should receive accessible education about menstrual hygiene and reproductive health. Caregivers and educators should ensure that information is provided in formats that suit individual needs, such as visual aids or simplified language.

Schools can be vital for delivering health education and services to girls with disabilities. These programs should be inclusive and adaptable. Teaching girls about their rights as patients empowers them to advocate for better care. Parents and caregivers can also play an active role in advocating for improved healthcare access. Inclusive programs that integrate girls with disabilities into community or school activities help reduce stigma and foster supportive environments.

Creating a supportive environment for girls with chronic conditions and disabilities involves collaboration between families, educators, healthcare providers, and communities. We can help these girls lead fulfilling lives and achieve their potential by addressing their physical, emotional, and social needs.

The future of health equity depends on recognizing and addressing the unique challenges girls face. Through tailored care, education, and advocacy, we can ensure that every girl has the opportunity to thrive, regardless of her health condition or disability.

Did you know?

- *Girls with diabetes who learn self-management skills early—such as checking blood sugar and understanding nutrition—are more likely to maintain healthy long-term outcomes and experience fewer hospitalizations.*
- *Girls with disabilities are at a higher risk of overlooked health issues, like osteoporosis or untreated pain, simply because routine screenings are often missed. Inclusive healthcare practices can dramatically reduce these risks and improve quality of life.*

Body and External Genital Hygiene: Nurturing Healthy Habits from Childhood

Hygiene is not merely a routine but a foundation for good health and well-being, instilled in early childhood and carried throughout life. For young girls, learning proper hygiene practices goes beyond cleanliness; it shapes their confidence and helps them build a positive relationship with their bodies.

From birth, a child's skin requires attentive care. Soft and sensitive, it is prone to irritation, redness, and inflammation, particularly in areas exposed to moisture, such as the perineal and anal regions. This is especially true for children wearing diapers, where prolonged exposure to dampness can cause discomfort and rashes. Parents can prevent these issues by gently wiping the area with wet wipes during every diaper change and washing the child with warm water after defecation. These early routines form the building blocks of lifelong hygiene habits.

As infants grow, they may develop white secretions or a thin film in the folds of the labia minora, labia majora, and groin. While this can alarm parents, these secretions are natural and do not require harsh cleaning or aggressive removal. A daily rinse with warm water suffices for infants, and soap should only be used sparingly, perhaps every other day. Parents should avoid fragranced soaps and body washes when choosing products, opting instead for gentle baby soap. The direction of washing, constantly moving from the pubic area toward the anus, further ensures cleanliness without spreading bacteria.

After washing, the perineal area should be gently dried with a soft towel. To prevent cross-contamination, the individual should use towels exclusively and explicitly designated for intimate hygiene. Parents must teach these practices early, making them second nature to their children. This individualized approach to hygiene not only prevents infections but also reinforces the importance of self-care.

Bathing is often a source of joy for young children. The warm water and bubbles transform cleanliness into a moment of play and relaxation. However, certain precautions ensure that this cherished ritual remains beneficial. To protect sensitive skin, the water temperature should be comfortably warm, never hot. While foaming agents and bath additives may be tempting, they should be used sparingly, as prolonged contact with foam can irritate the external genitalia, causing itching or burning.

As children mature, transitioning from baths to showers becomes essential to their hygiene routine. Showers are generally more hygienic, as they reduce prolonged exposure to potentially irritating substances. Even after a bath, a quick rinse under the shower can remove any lingering soap or foam, ensuring thorough cleanliness. Practices such as sitz baths and douching, which can disrupt the delicate balance of the skin and reproductive system, should be avoided altogether for both children and adults.

The role of clothing in hygiene cannot be overstated, particularly when it comes to underwear. Clean, comfortable undergarments made of natural materials such as cotton or silk allow the skin to breathe and reduce the risk of irritation or infection. Washing underwear separately from other clothing with mild, eco-friendly detergents further minimizes the likelihood of allergic reactions.

Teenagers, especially girls, may adopt habits such as using disposable panty liners. While these can offer convenience, they should never replace the essential practice of changing underwear daily. Fashion trends like thong underwear often spark debate, but they pose no inherent risk when properly sized and worn appropriately. However, they serve little functional purpose beyond aesthetics, making traditional options more practical for everyday wear.

The onset of menstruation marks a transformative phase in a girl's life, requiring a heightened focus on hygiene. Washing the external genital area twice daily, once in the morning and once in the evening, becomes particularly important. For girls who choose tampons, it is recommended to limit their use to daytime hours, as overnight use can increase the risk of complications such as toxic shock syndrome. Sanitary pads remain a safer option for nighttime protection.

Menstrual hygiene education allows parents to address broader aspects of self-care and sexual health, laying the groundwork for informed and responsible choices in the future.

Hair removal in intimate areas has become increasingly popular among teenagers and women. While various methods are available, ranging from professional treatments to at-home solutions, the choice often depends on personal preference and resources. For teenagers, guidance from a parent, particularly a mother, can be invaluable in selecting a safe and suitable method for their age. Razors, if used, should always be personal and never shared to prevent the spread of infections.

Beyond hair removal, allowing the perineal area to breathe is essential. Tight clothing that compresses the abdomen and thighs should be avoided as it limits air circulation, leading to discomfort and irritation.

Nightwear is a personal choice shaped by individual preferences and habits. Whether a girl sleeps in pajamas, a nightgown, or without clothing, the key considerations remain the same: the attire should be loose-fitting to prevent overheating and changed regularly to maintain cleanliness. Comfortable nightwear contributes to restful sleep, supporting overall health and well-being.

Teaching hygiene is a fundamental aspect of parenting, as vital as feeding, education, and emotional support. Hygiene practices must evolve alongside a child's growth, addressing the changing needs of their body. Parents play an indispensable role in fostering a positive attitude toward self-care by creating an open and supportive environment where questions are welcomed, and guidance is readily available.

By instilling these practices from an early age, parents protect their children from potential health issues and empower them to take pride in their personal hygiene. This foundation of care and attention ensures that girls grow up with the knowledge and confidence to maintain their health and well-being.

Did You Know?

- *The Direction of Washing Matters: Always wash from the pubic area toward the anus to avoid spreading bacteria and reduce the risk of urinary or genital infections.*
- *Panty Liners Have Limits: Disposable panty liners can be convenient but should never replace the daily practice of changing underwear, which is essential for maintaining hygiene.*

The Role of Fathers in a Girl's Growth, Success, and Health

The relationship between a father and his daughter is a cornerstone of her emotional and psychological development. Fathers play a pivotal role in shaping a girl's self-esteem, resilience, and understanding of the world. Their influence extends beyond childhood, leaving lasting impressions on how daughters perceive themselves, navigate relationships, and approach challenges in life. Recognizing the profound impact of fathers highlights the need for intentional, nurturing engagement throughout a girl's life.

A father's presence and involvement in his daughter's life provide an essential sense of security and emotional stability. For girls, having a reliable and supportive father figure fosters trust and confidence in forming relationships with others. Fathers who express love, encouragement, and respect establish a foundation for their daughters to feel valued and understood.

Girls often look to their fathers for affirmation. When a father validates his daughter's worth through words and actions, he contributes significantly to her self-esteem. Conversely, a lack of emotional connection or inconsistent support can lead to feelings of inadequacy or insecurity. The emotional bond between a father and daughter is especially critical during adolescence, a time when girls are navigating identity and self-worth. Fathers who remain attentive and present during this period can help mitigate the adverse effects of societal pressures, such as body image concerns and peer influences.

Fathers play an instrumental role in encouraging their daughters to explore their interests and embrace new opportunities. By supporting their passions and celebrating their achievements, fathers empower girls to develop independence and confidence. This encouragement often translates into academic, professional, and personal success.

A father's belief in his daughter's abilities has a ripple effect, shaping her belief in herself. When fathers teach their daughters to approach challenges with determination and resilience, they foster a mindset of perseverance. Fathers who model problem-solving, critical thinking, and adaptability demonstrate the value of these skills, enabling their daughters to approach obstacles with courage and resourcefulness.

How a father interacts with his daughter and women in his life profoundly influences a girl's understanding of relationships. Fathers who demonstrate respect, kindness, and equality in their interactions set a standard for how their daughters expect to be treated by others. These examples help girls develop healthy boundaries and recognize positive relationship dynamics.

Conversely, hostile behaviors such as neglect, criticism, or aggression can shape unhealthy patterns in a girl's relationships. Fathers must be mindful of their actions and words, as daughters often internalize these moments. Fathers who engage in open, respectful communication with their daughters create a safe environment for discussing feelings, experiences, and concerns, laying the groundwork for trust and mutual understanding.

A father's influence extends to his daughter's physical and mental health. Fathers who encourage active lifestyles, balanced nutrition, and regular exercise contribute to their daughters' overall well-being. These habits, instilled early, often carry into adulthood, promoting long-term health benefits.

A father's involvement equally impacts mental health. Fathers who prioritize open dialogue about emotions and mental well-being help normalize conversations about mental health. This openness reduces stigma and encourages daughters to seek support when needed. Additionally, fathers who model stress management and emotional regulation provide their daughters with valuable tools for handling life's challenges.

Girls often face societal expectations that can be limiting or damaging. Fathers have the unique opportunity to challenge these norms by advocating for their daughters' rights and aspirations. When fathers actively support their daughters' ambitions, regardless of traditional gender roles, they reinforce the message that girls can achieve anything they want.

For example, a father's encouragement in traditionally male-dominated fields, such as science, technology, engineering, and mathematics (STEM), can inspire a daughter to pursue her interests without fear of bias or discrimination. Fathers who champion gender equality in their homes and communities help dismantle stereotypes, creating a more inclusive environment for their daughters to thrive.

The relationship between a father and daughter is not static; it evolves. Fathers who remain engaged and adaptive as their daughters grow foster enduring connections. From playful interactions during childhood to meaningful conversations in adolescence and adulthood, the bond between a father and daughter deepens with shared experiences and mutual respect.

Fathers should prioritize quality time with their daughters, listening actively and participating in activities that strengthen their relationship. Simple gestures, such as attending school events, celebrating milestones, or sharing hobbies, create lasting memories and reinforce the importance of their bond.

The role of fathers in a girl's life cannot be overstated. Their involvement shapes her emotional resilience, confidence, and understanding of the world. Fathers prioritizing love, respect, and encouragement give their daughters the tools to succeed and thrive in every aspect of life. By embracing their unique role, fathers have the power to positively influence their daughters and future generations of women who will carry their legacy forward.

Did you know?

- *A father's encouragement and belief in his daughter's abilities significantly boost her self-esteem, resilience, and confidence. This support often translates into more tremendous success in academic, professional, and personal pursuits.*
- *Fathers who model respect, kindness, and equality in their relationships set a powerful example for their daughters, shaping their expectations for healthy relationships and*

empowering them to establish firm boundaries and positive dynamics.

Your Child's Health Is in Your Hands

To everyone who took the time to read this book, thank you. I hope it has provided you with valuable insights and tools to care for your child thoughtfully and informedly.

Being a parent is one of life's most challenging yet rewarding roles. It demands accountability and attentiveness that shape the lives of those who rely on us for their growth, security, and happiness. Unlike many roles in life, parenting does not come with a manual, and it doesn't grant us the option to choose our children. Instead, we create them through our actions, our words, and the environments we nurture.

But remember that the "finished product" is not the fragile newborn we cradle in our arms. It is the person they grow into over years of learning, guidance, and support. The essence of parenting lies in shaping a healthy child and a resilient individual who steps into adulthood with confidence, empathy, and the ability to navigate an ever-changing world.

Children reflect the lives of the adults who surround them. Their physical health is often a direct consequence of how we care for their bodies, and their emotional well-being mirrors the dynamics of our relationships. The joy and love we bring into their lives leave a lasting imprint, just as stress, anger, or neglect can leave scars.

This means that our children's physical, mental, and emotional health depends heavily on our own. We must strive to model the behaviors we hope they will adopt, fostering habits of kindness, self-care, and curiosity. The environment we create in our homes, the emotions we display, and the priorities we uphold serve as their blueprint for engaging with the world.

"*Nature wants children to be children before they are adults. Let childhood mature within them*," wrote Jean-Jacques Rousseau. These words are a timeless reminder of letting children live as children. Their early years are precious and fleeting, a period of wonder, exploration, and innocence that should be protected and cherished.

If you carry joyful childhood memories, let those moments inspire you to create the same for your children. If challenges marked your childhood, remember that you can break cycles and provide something better for the next generation.

Children need not perfection but love, presence, and understanding. They will not remember every gift you gave them or every detail of your efforts. They will remember how you made them feel safe, supported, and deeply loved.

Parenting does not require us to have all the answers. It asks only that we try, every day, to meet our children with compassion, patience, and an open heart. There will be mistakes and moments of uncertainty, but these are part of the journey.

Above all, love your children. Show them, in your words and actions, that they are valued. And as you nurture their growth, remember to promote yourself, for your health and happiness are intricately tied to theirs.

Thank you for joining me on this journey. May the insights in this book guide you as you care for your children and, in doing so, shape a future full of possibility and hope.

Love your children.

Olena Berezovska

Vocabulary of terms and conceptions

A

- Acyclic Pain: Pelvic pain that occurs at any time during the menstrual cycle, not just during menstruation.
- Acne: A chronic inflammatory condition of the hair follicles and sebaceous glands, characterized by pimples, blackheads, and cysts, often linked to hormonal changes.
- ADHD (Attention Deficit Hyperactivity Disorder): A neurodevelopmental disorder marked by inattention, hyperactivity, and impulsivity, more commonly diagnosed in boys.
- Adolescent Hormonal Fluctuations: Hormonal changes during puberty that influence mood, behavior, and physical appearance.
- Adolescent Pregnancy: Pregnancy occurring in girls aged 10–19 years is often associated with higher risks due to physical and emotional immaturity.
- Adrenarche: The rise in adrenal androgens, such as DHEA and androstenedione, marking the early hormonal phase of puberty.
- Amenorrhea: Absence of menstruation, often caused by nutritional deficiencies, excessive physical activity, or stress.
- Amniocentesis: A procedure where amniotic fluid is extracted to analyze fetal chromosomes.
- Amygdala: A brain structure involved in emotions, particularly fear, aggression, and processing threats. It develops earlier in boys, influencing their action-oriented responses to emotions.
- Anemia: A condition marked by a deficiency of red blood cells or hemoglobin, leading to fatigue and pale skin.
- Anovulation: The absence of ovulation during a menstrual cycle, often leading to irregular or missed periods.

- Androgens: Hormones primarily associated with male traits, such as testosterone, promote muscle growth, deep voices, and sperm production.
- Antifibrinolytics: Medications that prevent the breakdown of blood clots, commonly prescribed for treating bleeding disorders.
- Antifungal Creams: Topical medications used to treat fungal infections by inhibiting fungal growth.
- Apoptosis: A natural process of programmed cell death, contributing to breast discomfort as tissue cells are shed during the menstrual cycle.
- Autonomous Nervous System: Part of the nervous system that regulates involuntary body functions, including those of the pelvic organs.
- Autism Spectrum Disorder (ASD): A developmental condition affecting communication, behavior, and social interactions, with gender-based symptom differences.
- Autosomes: Chromosomes that do not determine sex but carry other genetic information.
- AUB (Abnormal Uterine Bleeding): Bleeding from the uterus that occurs outside of the normal menstrual cycle.
- Axillary Hair: Hair that grows in the underarm region, commonly appearing during puberty.

B

- Basal Layer: The deeper layer of the endometrium from which new tissue regenerates after menstruation.
- Benign: Non-cancerous; describes a mass or tumor that does not spread to other body parts.
- Biopsychosocial Model: A holistic framework categorizing health determinants into biological, psychological, and social factors.
- Body Dysmorphic Disorder (BDD): A mental health condition characterized by obsessive focus on perceived physical flaws.
- Body Image: A person's perception and attitude toward their physical appearance.

- Bone Age: A measure of skeletal maturity compared to chronological age, often advanced in cases of precocious puberty.
- Bone Mineral Density (BMD): A bone strength measure often reduced by hormonal imbalances or poor nutrition.
- Brain Blood Flow refers to the circulation of blood within the brain, which delivers oxygen and nutrients. Girls have more central blood flow, while boys have higher peripheral blood flow.
- Breast Buds: The first visible sign of puberty in girls, marking the beginning of breast development.
- Breast Swelling: Temporary enlargement of breast tissue in newborns due to maternal hormonal influence.
- Breastfeeding: Feeding an infant with breast milk provides essential nutrients and immunity support.
- Breathable Clothing: Attire that allows for adequate air circulation, reducing discomfort and the risk of skin irritation in intimate areas.
- Breast Tissue: The glandular and fatty tissue in the chest that develops during puberty and varies in size and shape.

C

- Calcium Metabolism: The body's process of absorbing and utilizing calcium, essential for maintaining strong bones.
- Cartilage Piercing: A piercing in harder tissue, which heals more slowly and is prone to infections.
- Cervical Mucus: Fluid secreted by the cervix that changes in consistency during the menstrual cycle, aiding or hindering sperm movement.
- Cervix: The lower part of the uterus, connecting to the vagina.
- Chromosomes: Structures within cells containing genetic information. Humans typically have 46 chromosomes, including two sex chromosomes.
- Circadian Rhythms: The 24-hour biological cycles that regulate sleep, activity, and other physiological processes.

- Clitoromegaly: Enlargement of the clitoris, often temporary in newborns exposed to maternal hormones.
- Coagulopathies: Disorders impairing blood clotting, contributing to excessive bleeding.
- Combined Oral Contraceptives (COCs): Hormonal medications containing estrogen and progesterone are often used to regulate menstrual cycles or treat heavy bleeding.
- Comedones: Skin blemishes that form when hair follicles are clogged with oil and dead skin cells. Open comedones are blackheads, and closed comedones are whiteheads.
- Consent: Voluntary agreement to participate in an activity central to healthy relationships and the prevention of sexual violence.
- Contraception: Methods or devices used to prevent pregnancy, including hormonal, barrier, and emergency options.
- Corpus Callosum: A structure connecting the left and right brain hemispheres, facilitating communication between them.
- Corpus Luteum: A temporary ovarian structure formed after ovulation that produces progesterone.
- Cortisol: A stress hormone produced by the adrenal glands. Girls tend to have higher cortisol sensitivity, making them more prone to stress-related anxiety.

D

- Deadnaming: Referring to a transgender person by their birth name after they have adopted a new name.
- Delayed Puberty (DP): Absence of pubertal signs by age 13–14 or a failure to menstruate within five years after breast development begins.
- Dermis: The deeper layer of skin where tattoo ink is injected, making tattoos permanent.
- Digital Bystanders: Individuals who observe or indirectly participate in cyberviolence by sharing, liking, or ignoring harmful content.

- Digital Literacy: The ability to navigate, evaluate, and communicate effectively online.
- Dyslexia: A learning disorder affecting reading and language processing. It is more common in boys and is often linked to differences in brain structure.
- Dysmenorrhea: Painful menstruation, often involving abdominal cramps.
- Dysplasia: Abnormal growth or development of cells, often detected in the cervix during screening tests.

E

- Ecological Systems Theory: A model developed by Urie Bronfenbrenner explaining how interactions within multiple environmental layers influence a child's development.
- Emergency Contraception: Methods used after unprotected intercourse to prevent pregnancy, such as high-dose progestins or IUDs.
- Endocrine-disrupting chemicals (EDCs) are substances, like bisphenol A (BPA) and phthalates, that interfere with the hormonal system and can impact puberty and reproductive health.
- Endometriosis: A condition where tissue similar to the uterine lining grows outside the uterus, causing pain and potential infertility.
- Endometrium: The inner lining of the uterus thickens during the menstrual cycle to prepare for pregnancy and sheds during menstruation.
- Empowerment: Increasing confidence and control over one's decisions and actions, often through education and skill-building.
- Epigenetics: The study of how environmental factors influence gene activity without altering the DNA sequence.
- Estriol: A type of estrogen produced in high amounts during pregnancy.
- Estrogen: A primary female sex hormone that regulates reproductive functions and contributes to emotional

connectivity, fat distribution, and skeletal maturation in girls.

- Exosystem: External environments that indirectly affect a child, such as a parent's workplace or local government policies.

F

- Family History: The medical history of a patient's relatives is significant for evaluating the likelihood of hereditary conditions.
- Female Athlete Triad: A syndrome involving energy deficiency, menstrual dysfunction, and decreased bone density.
- Ferriman-Gallwey Scoring System: A scale used to measure the severity of hirsutism based on hair growth in specific areas of the body.
- Fine Motor Skills: Movements involving small muscle groups, such as writing or drawing. These skills develop earlier in girls.
- Functional Ovarian Cysts: Fluid-filled sacs forming in the ovaries, often resolving without treatment.

G

- Gender Dysphoria: Distress due to a mismatch between one's gender identity and assigned sex at birth.
- Gender Identity: A person's deeply felt sense of being male, female, or somewhere on the gender spectrum.
- Gonads: The reproductive organs (testes in males, ovaries in females) responsible for producing sex cells and hormones.
- Gonadotropins: Hormones produced by the pituitary gland that stimulate the ovaries to produce eggs and sex hormones.
- Grooming: A process where predators build trust with a victim to facilitate exploitation.
- Gross Motor Skills: Movements involving large muscle groups, such as running or jumping.

H

- Heavy Menstrual Bleeding (HMB): Excessive blood loss during menstruation that interferes with daily activities.
- Hormonal Balance: The equilibrium of hormones in the body, essential for maintaining normal physiological functions.
- Hormonal Contraceptives: Medications containing hormones like estrogen and progesterone to regulate cycles or prevent pregnancy.
- Hormones: Chemical messengers produced by glands that influence development, growth, and reproduction.
- Human Papillomavirus (HPV): A viral infection that can cause genital warts and is associated with cervical cancer. Vaccines are available to prevent infection.
- Hyperandrogenism: A condition characterized by elevated androgen levels in women, leading to symptoms such as acne, hirsutism, or hair thinning.
- Hypothalamic-Pituitary-Gonadal Axis (HPG Axis): The hormonal system involving the hypothalamus, pituitary gland, and gonads (ovaries or testes), which regulate puberty and reproductive function.
- Hypothalamus: A small region at the base of the brain that plays a crucial role in regulating various physiological processes, including temperature control, hunger, thirst, sleep, emotional responses, and the release of hormones via the pituitary gland.
- Hypothyroidism: A condition in which the thyroid gland produces insufficient hormones, often leading to symptoms like fatigue, weight gain, and heavy menstrual bleeding.

I

- Infertility: A condition in which a couple is unable to conceive after one year of regular, unprotected intercourse.
- Intrauterine Device (IUD): A small, T-shaped device inserted into the uterus to prevent pregnancy.
- Insulin Resistance: A condition where the body's cells do not respond effectively to insulin, often linked to PCOS and an increased risk of type 2 diabetes.

- Intense Pulsed Light (IPL): A cosmetic treatment using light to reduce hair density and improve skin appearance.

J

- Juvenile Uterine Bleeding: A subtype of abnormal uterine bleeding specific to adolescents, often related to the immaturity of the reproductive system.

K

- Karyotype: The complete set of chromosomes in an individual used to identify genetic abnormalities.
- Keloid: An overgrown scar that can form after a piercing or tattoo, particularly in individuals prone to such conditions.
- Keratin: A structural protein in skin, hair, and nails, providing strength and resilience.
- Ketogenic Diet: A high-fat, low-carbohydrate diet sometimes used to manage weight or treat specific medical conditions.

L

- Labiaplasty: Surgical reshaping or reduction of the labia minora, often performed for aesthetic or functional purposes.
- Laparoscopy: A minimally invasive surgical procedure used to diagnose or treat conditions such as endometriosis or ovarian cysts.
- Laser Tattoo Removal: A method using high-intensity lasers to break down tattoo ink for gradual elimination by the body.
- Luteal Phase: The second phase of the menstrual cycle occurs after ovulation, during which the uterine lining prepares for the possible implantation of a fertilized egg.
- Luteinizing Hormone (LH): A hormone produced by the pituitary gland that stimulates ovulation and ovarian hormone production.
- Lactation: The process of producing and secreting milk from the mammary glands to feed an infant.

- Leukorrhea: A mild, whitish vaginal discharge that is common during different stages of the menstrual cycle or pregnancy.
- Lifestyle Medicine: A medical approach focusing on diet, exercise, and behavioral changes to prevent and treat chronic conditions.

M

- Macrosystem: A child's overall environment is influenced by the larger societal and cultural context, including norms, laws, and economic conditions.
- Malignant: Cancerous; describes a mass or tumor that can invade surrounding tissues or spread to other body areas.
- Mammography: A screening tool that uses X-rays to detect abnormalities in breast tissue, often used to identify early signs of breast cancer.
- Mastalgia: Breast pain or tenderness, often linked to hormonal fluctuations during the menstrual cycle.
- Menarche: The first occurrence of menstruation in a girl's life, marking the onset of reproductive capability.
- Menorrhagia: Abnormally heavy or prolonged menstrual bleeding.
- Menstrual hygiene uses pads, tampons, or cups to manage menstrual bleeding while maintaining cleanliness and health.
- Metabolic Syndrome: A cluster of conditions, including insulin resistance, obesity, and high cholesterol, increasing the risk of heart disease and diabetes.
- Microbiome: The collection of microorganisms, including bacteria and fungi, that live in or on the human body, influencing health and disease.
- Multitasking: The ability to perform multiple tasks simultaneously. Girls are more adept due to larger corpus callosum development, enabling better communication between brain hemispheres.

N

- Neuroplasticity: The brain's ability to adapt and change through experience, underpinning learning and development.
- Nonsteroidal Anti-Inflammatory Drugs (NSAIDs): Medications like ibuprofen that reduce inflammation and pain are often used to manage heavy menstrual bleeding and dysmenorrhea.
- Nipple Discharge: Fluid secretion from the nipple may range from clear or milky (typically harmless) to colored or bloody, requiring medical evaluation.
- Nightwear Hygiene: Wear clean, loose-fitting clothing or sleeping unclothed to promote rest and avoid overheating.
- Neuroendocrine System: The interaction between the nervous system and the endocrine system in regulating bodily functions, including puberty and reproduction.
- Nutritional Deficiency: A lack of essential nutrients in the diet, which can lead to conditions like anemia, delayed puberty, or weakened immunity.

O

- Oligomenorrhea: Menstrual cycles longer than 35 days are standard in adolescents due to the immaturity of the hypothalamic-pituitary-ovarian axis.
- Oral Contraceptives: Pills containing hormones that prevent ovulation and are used for birth control or to regulate menstrual cycles.
- Osteoporosis: A condition characterized by weak and brittle bones, often influenced by hormonal changes and nutrient deficiencies.
- Ovarian Cysts: Fluid-filled sacs that form on or in the ovaries, often harmless but sometimes requiring medical attention.
- Ovulation: The release of a mature egg from the ovary, typically occurring monthly after puberty.
- Oxytocin: A hormone associated with bonding, attachment, and stress reduction.

P

- Pap Smear: A test that collects cervical cells to detect abnormalities, precancerous changes, or infections.
- Pelvic Inflammatory Disease (PID): An infection of the uterus, fallopian tubes, or ovaries, often caused by untreated STIs, which can lead to pain, infertility, or other complications.
- Placenta: The organ that connects the fetus to the uterine wall, providing oxygen, nutrients, and waste removal.
- Polycystic Ovary Syndrome (PCOS): A hormonal disorder characterized by irregular cycles, excessive hair growth, obesity, and polycystic ovaries.
- Postpartum Period: The six weeks after childbirth when the body recovers and adjusts hormonally and physically.
- Premature Adrenarche: Early growth of pubic or underarm hair caused by elevated androgen levels.
- Premature Thelarche: Early breast development, typically before age 3, without other signs of puberty.
- Premenstrual Syndrome (PMS): A group of symptoms, including mood swings, bloating, and fatigue, occurring in the luteal phase of the menstrual cycle.
- Primary Dysmenorrhea: Painful menstrual cramps caused by uterine contractions, not linked to underlying medical conditions.
- Progesterone: A hormone produced by the ovaries after ovulation, essential for regulating the menstrual cycle and supporting pregnancy.
- Prolactin: A hormone the pituitary gland produces, primarily involved in milk production during breastfeeding.
- Puberty: The biological stage of development during which sexual maturity is reached, marked by physical and hormonal changes.

R

- Reproductive Health: Physical, mental, and social well-being in matters related to the reproductive system at all stages of life.

- Retinoids: Vitamin A derivatives are often used to treat skin conditions like acne.
- Rickets: A condition in children caused by vitamin D deficiency, leading to weak or soft bones and skeletal deformities.
- Rumination Disorder: A rare condition where individuals regurgitate food repeatedly, re-chewing and sometimes re-swallowing it.

S

- Secondary Sexual Characteristics: Physical traits that develop during puberty, such as breast growth and body hair, distinguish males from females.
- Spermicides: Chemical substances that kill sperm to prevent fertilization.
- Steroid Hormones: A family of hormones derived from cholesterol, including sex hormones and adrenal hormones.
- Suprapubic Pain: Pain above the pubic bone, commonly associated with bladder or lower intestinal conditions.
- Synthetic Progestins: Lab-created forms of the hormone progesterone regulate menstrual cycles or treat heavy bleeding.

T

- Tanner Stages: A classification system for the progression of physical changes during puberty, ranging from Stage 1 (prepubertal) to Stage 5 (full maturity).
- Testosterone: A primary male sex hormone that influences muscle growth, risk-taking behaviors, and spatial skills.
- Thelarche: The first stage of breast development, marked by the formation of breast buds.
- Toxic Shock Syndrome (TSS): A rare but serious condition caused by certain bacterial infections, often associated with improper tampon use.
- Transgender: A term describing individuals whose gender identity differs from the sex they were assigned at birth.

U

- Ultrasound: A non-invasive imaging technique that uses sound waves to create pictures of internal organs.
- Urinary Tract Infection (UTI): An infection affecting the bladder, urethra, or kidneys, more common in females due to their shorter urethra.
- Uterus: The hollow muscular organ in females where a fertilized egg implants and develops into a fetus.

V

- Vaccination: Administration of a vaccine to protect against infections, such as HPV and hepatitis B.
- Vestibule of the Vagina: The region within the vulva containing the vaginal and urethral openings.
- Virilization: A condition characterized by masculine physical traits in women, such as deepening of the voice or clitoral enlargement.
- Vulva: The external female genitalia, including the labia, clitoris, and vaginal opening.

W

- Withdrawal Bleeding: Menstrual-like bleeding that occurs after stopping hormonal contraception.

Y

- Yolk Sac: An embryonic structure where primary sex cells originate before migrating to the gonads.

Z

- Zygote: A fertilized egg cell resulting from the union of a sperm and an egg, representing the earliest stage of human development.

List of references

1. Al-Qaraghouli M, Villar J. Effect of fetal sex on maternal and obstetric outcomes. Front Pediatr. 2017;5:144.
2. Alrousan G. Early-life sleep deprivation highly influences future affective and behavioral problems. Pediatr Res. 2022;91(4):912-920.
3. American Academy of Pediatrics. Evidence-informed milestones for developmental surveillance tools. Pediatrics. 2022;149(3):e2021052138.
4. Bacaro V, et al. A meta-analysis of longitudinal studies on the interplay between sleep, mental health, and wellbeing in adolescents. Sleep Med Rev. 2024;65:101426.
5. Baines KJ, et al. Sex differences in innate and adaptive immunity impact fetal development. Placenta. 2023;137:26-34.
6. Balasundaram P. Human growth velocity during infancy and adolescence; patterns of height and weight changes. StatPearls. 2023.
7. Barker DJP, Osmond C. Infant mortality, childhood nutrition, and ischaemic heart disease in England and Wales. Lancet. 1986;327(8489):1077-1081.
8. Berger AT. Adolescent sleep epidemic: relationships between sleep duration and adolescent mental health. Sleep Health. 2019;5(4):362-367.
9. Bhutta ZA, Lassi ZS, Bergeron G, et al. Delivering an action agenda for nutrition interventions addressing adolescent girls and young women: priorities for the next decade. BMJ. 2021;373:n1403.
10. Biddle SJH. Physical activity and mental health in children and adolescents: overview of reviews. J Public Health (Oxf). 2019;27(Suppl 2):100-107.
11. Blum RW, Astone NM, Decker MR, Mouli VC. A conceptual framework for early adolescence: a platform for research. Int J Adolesc Med Health. 2014;26(3):321-331.

12. Camlin NJ, et al. Inhibition of WNT/β-catenin signalling during sex-specific development in human fetal gonads. Cell Commun Signal. 2024;22:34.
13. Capra ME, et al. Nutrition for children and adolescents who practice sport: a narrative review. Nutrients. 2024;16(16):2803.
14. Casey BJ, Jones RM, Hare TA. The adolescent brain. Ann N Y Acad Sci. 2008;1124(1):111-126.
15. Choudhury S, et al. Social cognitive development during adolescence. Soc Cogn Affect Neurosci. 2006;1(3):165-174.
16. Coast E. Puberty and menstruation knowledge among young females aged 10-14 years in low- and middle-income countries: a scoping review. PLoS One. 2019;14(5):e0216843.
17. Coledam DHC. Objective analysis of physical activity volume and intensity associated with adolescent mental health. J Public Health (Oxf). 2023;15(4):300-310.
18. Coledam DHC. Physical activity intensity thresholds and anxiety reduction in adolescents. Ment Health Phys Act. 2023;22:100-110.
19. Coledam DHC. Role of physical activity volume and intensity on adolescent mental health. Front Public Health. 2023;11:1150-1162.
20. Costello EJ, et al. Trends in psychopathology across the adolescent years: what changes when children become adolescents, and when adolescents become adults? J Child Psychol Psychiatry. 2011;52(10):1015-1025.
21. Cueto-Martín B, et al. Family influence on adolescent physical activity: a mediation model. Front Sports Act Living. 2024;6:1372664.
22. Dahl RE, et al. Importance of investing in adolescence from a developmental science perspective. Nature. 2018;554(7693):441-450.
23. Darabi F, et al. Effectiveness of pubertal and menstrual health education on health behaviors among Iranian

secondary school girls. J Prev Med Public Health. 2022;55(10):595-610.
24. Dick B, Ferguson BJ. Health for the world's adolescents: a second chance in the second decade. J Adolesc Health. 2015;56(1):3-6.
25. Ding D, et al. Built environment's influence on adolescent physical activity and mental health. Am J Prev Med. 2021;61(3):310-318.
26. Ding D, et al. Physical activity behaviors in adolescence: evidence and intervention opportunities. Lancet Child Adolesc Health. 2021;5(3):190-200.
27. DiPietro JA. The gestational foundation of sex differences in development and vulnerability. Neurosci Biobehav Rev. 2010;35(1):56-64.
28. Evans RL. Systematic review of educational interventions to improve menstrual knowledge, attitudes, and practices. BMJ Open. 2022;12(6):e057204.
29. Gao M, et al. Sleep duration and depression among adolescents: mediation effect of collective integration. Front Psychol. 2022;13:101508.
30. Garcia-Alonso L, et al. Deciphering sex-specific differentiation of human fetal gonads using single-cell transcriptomics. Front Cell Dev Biol. 2022;10:902082.
31. Gauchat A. Poor sleep correlates with externalizing and internalizing behavior problems in children. Front Neurol. 2020;11:624.
32. Gbogbo S. Menstrual health needs and educational outcomes among adolescent girls: a systematic review. Public Health Rev. 2025;47(3):200-215.
33. Engel GL. The need for a new medical model: a challenge for biomedicine. Science. 1977;196(4286):129-136.
34. Giedd JN. The teen brain: insights from neuroimaging. J Adolesc Health. 2008;42(4):335-343.
35. Gilchrist JD. Effects of reallocating physical activity, sedentary behaviors, and sleep on adolescent mental health. Sleep. 2021;44(8):zsab111.

36. Gualdi-Russo E, et al. Physical activity and body image perception in adolescents: a systematic review. Int J Environ Res Public Health. 2022;19(20):13190.
37. Haberland NA. A systematic review of adolescent girl programs: health and wellbeing outcomes in LMICs. J Adolesc Health. 2018;63(4):S21-S22.
38. Hale GE. Physical activity decline and its impact on adolescent psychological health: a review. Child Adolesc Ment Health. 2021;26(4):265-274.
39. Halfon N, et al. Life course health development: past, present, and future. Matern Child Health J. 2013;17(2):344-365.
40. Hayley AC, et al. Symptoms of depression and difficulty initiating sleep from early adolescence to young adulthood: a longitudinal study. Sleep. 2015;38(10):1599-1608.
41. Head A, Cheng M, Manica S. Effectiveness of menstrual health interventions in East Asia and the Pacific: a systematic review. Int J Environ Res Public Health. 2024;21(4):321-338.
42. Herbert AC. Puberty experiences of low-income girls in the United States: a systematic review. J Adolesc Health. 2017;61(3):294-300.
43. Heslin AM. Adolescent nutrition and health: characteristics, risk factors, and overlooked life-stage challenges. Nutrients. 2023;82(2):142-156.
44. Hjern A. Systematic review of prevention and treatment of infantile colic. Acta Paediatr. 2020;109(12):2362-2370.
45. Hosokawa R, Katsura T. Parental support for physical activity and children's behavior. Sci Rep. 2023;13(1):4572.
46. Hoyt LT. Timing of puberty in boys and girls: implications for health sequelae. Curr Opin Pediatr. 2020;32(4):509-515.
47. Huang X, et al. Family communication and adolescent mental health: mediating effects. BMC Public Health. 2023;23(1):16637.

48. Ibitoye M, et al. Early menarche: a systematic review of its effect on sexual and reproductive health in low- and middle-income countries. PLoS One. 2017;12(6):e0178884.
49. Kale R. "It's a girl!"—could be a death sentence. CMAJ. 2012;184(4):387.
50. Kamionka A, et al. Impact of parental attitudes on child physical activity. J Child Health. 2023;12(4):200-208.
51. Kessler RC, et al. Age of onset of mental disorders: a review of recent literature. Curr Opin Psychiatry. 2007;20(4):359-364.
52. Khor SPH, et al. Modifiable parental factors in adolescent sleep: a systematic review and meta-analysis. Sleep Med Rev. 2021;56:101408.
53. Kinnear HM, et al. Ovarian development and disease: the known and the unknown. Semin Cell Dev Biol. 2015;45:53-60.
54. Kokandakar AH. Sports participation type and adolescent self-rated health: longitudinal findings. J Adolesc Health. 2024;74(6):813-821.
55. Kwon EJ, Kim YJ. What is fetal programming: a lifetime of health is under the influence. Endocrinol Metab Clin North Am. 2017;46(2):243-256.
56. Lardon A, et al. Is puberty a risk factor for back pain in the young? A systematic critical literature review. Spine J. 2014;22:27-35.
57. Lassi ZS, et al. Effects of preventive nutrition interventions among adolescents on health and nutritional status in low- and middle-income countries: a systematic review and meta-analysis. Nutrients. 2020;12(1):49.
58. Lassi ZS, et al. Systematic review on evidence-based adolescent nutrition interventions. Ann N Y Acad Sci. 2017;1393(1):34-50.
59. Leung AKC. Gastroesophageal reflux in children: an updated review. Paediatr Drugs. 2019;21(4):281-291.

60. Liew SH, et al. The ovarian reserve is depleted during puberty in a hormonally driven process dependent on the proapoptotic protein BMF. Cell Death Dis. 2017;8:e2971.
61. Lindsay KL, et al. The interplay between maternal nutrition and stress in pregnancy: effects on fetal brain development. Rev Endocr Metab Disord. 2018;19(3):243-252.
62. Liu C. Physical activity interventions and mental health outcomes in children: a meta-analysis. JAMA Pediatr. 2024;178(5):455-462.
63. Lollies F. Sleep problems and sleep deprivation are associated with decreased functional emotion regulation and impaired emotion generation. J Sleep Res. 2022;31(6):e13621.
64. Lu B, et al. Global burden of depression or depressive symptoms in children and adolescents: a systematic review and meta-analysis. J Affect Disord. 2024;354:553-562.
65. Ludwig-Walz H. Dose-response relationship between lockdown severity and youth anxiety. Eur Child Adolesc Psychiatry. 2022;31(8):1191-1202.
66. MacDonald NE. Mandatory infant and childhood immunization: rationales and challenges. Vaccine. 2018;36(25):3593-3598.
67. Madigan S. Changes in depression and anxiety among children and adolescents during vs before COVID-19: systematic review and meta-analysis. JAMA Pediatr. 2023;177(2):166-177.
68. Madigan S. Long-term impact of pandemic on adolescent depression trajectories. Dev Psychol. 2023;59(7):1410-1422.
69. Man L, et al. Ovarian reserve disorders, can we prevent them? A review. Int J Mol Sci. 2022;23(23):15426.
70. Marciniak A, et al. Fetal programming of the metabolic syndrome. Clin Nutr. 2017;36(2):548-556.
71. Michaud PA, et al. The adolescent with a chronic condition. Part I: developmental issues. Arch Dis Child. 2007;92(11):938-942.

72. Mohapatra S. Global legal responses to prenatal gender identification. Indiana J Glob Leg Stud. 2013;20(2):489-512.
73. Moretti MM, Peled M. Adolescent–parent attachment and healthy adolescent functioning. Adolescence. 2004;39(153):519-534.
74. Murray GK, et al. Infant developmental milestones and subsequent intellectual outcomes. Br J Psychiatry. 2007;191(4):372-377.
75. Neumann CG, Alpaugh M. Infant birthweight doubling time: a fresh look. Pediatrics. 1976;57(4):469-473.
76. Nugent BM, et al. Placental H3K27me3 establishes female resilience to prenatal insults. Nat Commun. 2018;9(1):2555.
77. Patton GC, et al. Our future: a Lancet commission on adolescent health and wellbeing. Lancet. 2016;387(10036):2423-2478.
78. Patton GC, Temmerman M. Evidence and evidence gaps in adolescent health. J Adolesc Health. 2016;59(4 Suppl):S1-S3.
79. Paus T, et al. Why do many psychiatric disorders emerge during adolescence? Nat Rev Neurosci. 2008;9(12):947-957.
80. Petersen TL, et al. Parent–child physical activity correlation: a systematic review. Int J Behav Nutr Phys Act. 2020;17(1):75.
81. Poveda NE, et al. Associations of growth trajectories from birth through adolescence with adult body composition. Public Health Nutr. 2023;26(10):1918-1926.
82. Rapee RM. Anxiety disorders in children and adolescents: a summary of progress and directions. J Am Acad Child Adolesc Psychiatry. 2023;62(3):320-330.
83. Ratnapalan S, Cohen-Silver J. Management of infantile colic: a review. Clin Pediatr (Phila). 2009;48(1):14-18.
84. Reynaud E, et al. More and better sleep is associated with improved behavioral and cognitive outcomes in preschool children. Sleep Med Rev. 2019;47:42-51.

85. Reynaud E, et al. Preschool night-waking trajectories predict inattention/hyperactivity symptom trajectories. Sleep. 2019;42(2):zsy239.
86. Rogol AD, et al. Growth and pubertal development in children and adolescents: effects of diet and physical activity. Am J Clin Nutr. 2000;72(suppl):521S-528S.
87. Ruiz-Ranz E. Physical activity, exercise, and mental health of healthy adolescents: a recent review. Front Psychol. 2024;15:1250-1265.
88. Salam RA, et al. Interventions to improve adolescent nutrition: a systematic review and meta-analysis. J Adolesc Health. 2016;59(4 Suppl):S29-S39.
89. Samad N, et al. School-based healthy eating interventions for adolescents aged 10-19 years: an umbrella review. Nutrients. 2024;21(2):117.
90. Sawyer SM, et al. Platforms for delivering adolescent health actions. Lancet Child Adolesc Health. 2019;3(3):164-172.
91. Sawyer SM, et al. The age of adolescence. Lancet Child Adolesc Health. 2018;2(3):223-228.
92. Sekido R, Lovell-Badge R. Sry and SoxE genes: how they participate in mammalian sex determination. Bioessays. 2009;31(9):900-909.
93. Sisk CL, Foster DL. The neural basis of puberty and adolescence. Nat Neurosci. 2004;7(10):1040-1047.
94. Sood S. Teething myths and facts. J Clin Pediatr Dent. 2010;35(1):9-12.
95. Sutherland S, Brunwasser SM. Sex differences in vulnerability to prenatal stress: a review of the recent literature. Curr Psychiatry Rep. 2018;20(11):102.
96. Tarokh L, et al. Sleep in adolescence: physiology, cognition and mental health. Neurosci Biobehav Rev. 2016;70:182-188.
97. Uccella S, et al. Sleep deprivation and insomnia in adolescence: a longitudinal predictor of depression. J Clin Sleep Med. 2023;19(2):289-297.

98. Ulrich ND, et al. Ovarian reserve testing: a review of the options, their applications, and limitations. Clin Obstet Gynecol. 2019;62(2):265-274.
99. Bronfenbrenner U. The ecology of human development: experiments by nature and design. Cambridge, MA: Harvard University Press; 1979:1-348.
100. Bronfenbrenner U. Toward an experimental ecology of human development. Am Psychol. 1977;32(7):513-531.
101. Viswanathan M. Screening for anxiety in children and adolescents: a systematic review to inform USPSTF. JAMA. 2022;327(8):728-745.
102. Wainstock T, et al. Fetal sex modifies effects of prenatal stress exposure and adverse birth outcomes. Stress. 2015;18(1):49-56.
103. Wallace WHB, Kelsey TW. Human ovarian reserve from conception to the menopause. PLoS One. 2010;5(1):e8772.
104. Wang X, et al. Mechanisms of ovarian aging in women: a review. J Ovarian Res. 2023;16:67.
105. World Health Organization. Adolescent health epidemiology. Geneva: WHO; 2023. Technical Report Series No. 894.
106. Yang Y, et al. Early gonadal development and sex determination in mammals. Int J Mol Sci. 2022;23(14):7500.
107. Zaccagni L, Gualdi-Russo E. The impact of sports involvement on body image perception and ideals: a systematic review and meta-analysis. Int J Environ Res Public Health. 2023;20(6):5228.
108. Zhao D, et al. Gender differences in infant mortality and neonatal morbidity in mixed-gender twins. Sci Rep. 2017;7:8736.

Olena Berezovska's books

1. Мій шлях до істини. Березовська О.А. — 90 стор. Самовидав. Івано-Франківськ, Україна, 1996.
2. Интернет: Мифы и реальность заработка. Березовская Е.П. — 110 стр. Несколько онлайн-публикаций. Украина-Россия-Беларусь, 2000. (Ebook ISBN: 978-0-9867786-5-0)
3. Тысячиии... вопросов и ответов по гинекологии. Березовская Е.П. — 360 стр. Пресс-экспресс. Львов, Україна, 2008. (Print ISBN: 966-8360-08-7)
4. Ангел. Березовская Е.П. — 94 стр. Торонто, Канада, 2008. (Print ISBN: 978-1-997797-06-7, Ebook ISBN: 978-0-9867786-2-9)
5. День серебристого дождя. Березовская Е.П. — 107 стр. Торонто, Канада, 2008. (Ebook ISBN: 978-0-9867786-3-6)
6. Настольное пособие для беременных женщин. Березовская Е.П. — 400 стр. International Academy of Healthy Life. Канада-Украина, 2010. (Print ISBN: 978-0-9867786-1-2)
7. Подготовка к беременности. Березовская Е.П. — 200 стр. International Academy of Healthy Life. Канада-Украина, 2011. (Print ISBN: 978-0-9867786-0-5)
8. Гормонотерапия в акушерстве и гинекологии: иллюзии и реальность. Березовская Е.П. — 600 стр. International Academy of Healthy Life. Канада, 2013. (Ebook ISBN: 978-0-9867786-6-7)
9. 9 месяцев счастья. Настольное пособие для беременных женщин. Березовская Е.П. — 596 стр. ЭКСМО. Москва, Россия, 2015. (Print and Ebook ISBN: 978-5-699-80102-2)
10. Настільний посібник для вагітних. Березовська О.П. — 400 стор. Электронна версія. International Academy of Healthy Life. Торонто, Канада, 2016. (Ebook ISBN: 978-0-9867786-1-2)

11. Підготовка до вагітності. Березовська О.П. — 205 стор. Электронна версія. International Academy of Healthy Life. Торонто, Канада, 2016. (Print ISBN: 978-0-9867786-0-5)
12. Посібник для вагітних. Березовська О.П. — 392 стор. Манускрипт. Львів, Україна, 2016. (Print ISBN: 978-966-2400-55-7)
13. 1000 вопросов и ответов по гинекологии. Березовская Е.П. — 432 стр. ЭКСМО. Москва, Россия, 2017. (Print and Ebook ISBN: 978-5-699-80101-5)
14. Дочки-матери: Все, о чем вам не рассказывала ваша мама и чему стоит научить свою дочь. Березовская Е.П. — 288 стр. ЭКСМО. Москва, Россия, 2018. (Print and Ebook ISBN: 978-5-04-090021-3)
15. 9 місяців щастя. Березовська О.П. — 576 стор. BookChef. Київ, Україна, 2018. (Print and Ebook ISBN: 978-617-7559-18-3)
16. 9 месяцев счастья (второе издание). Настольное пособие для беременных женщин. Березовская Е.П. — 596 стр. ЭКСМО. Москва, Россия, 2019. (Print and Ebook ISBN: 978-5-04-098981-2)
17. Это все гормоны! Березовская Е.П. — 410 стр. ЭКСМО. Москва, Россия, 2019. (Print and Ebook ISBN: 978-5-04-101870-2)
18. Малыш, ты скоро? Березовская Е.П. — 384 стр. ЭКСМО. Москва, Россия, 2019. (Print and Ebook ISBN: 978-5-04-103359-0)
19. Когда ты будешь готова. Березовская Е.П. — 348 стр. ЭКСМО. Москва, Россия, 2020. (Print and Ebook ISBN: 978-5-04-116932-9)
20. Здравствуй, малыш. Березовская Е.П. — 320 стр. ЭКСМО. Москва, Россия, 2021. (Print and Ebook ISBN 978-5-04-121120-2)
21. Педіатрія: у 3-х т. Т. 3: підручник для студ. вищих мед. навч. закладів IV рівня акред. Катілов О., Варзарь А., Валіуліс А., Дмитрієв Д., та ін. — 656 стор. Нова Книга. Вінниця, Україна, 2022. (Print ISBN: 978-966-382-931-9)

22. 9 місяців щастя. Посібник для вагітних (оновлене й доповнене видання). Березовська О.П. — 624 стор. BookChef. Київ, Україна, 2023. (Print and Ebook ISBN: 978-617-548-122-6)
23. Коли тобі 35+. Як завагітніти й народити дитину. Березовська О.П. — 256 стор. BookChef. Київ, Україна, 2023. (Print and Ebook ISBN: 978-617-548-124-0)
24. Когда тебе 35+. Как забеременеть и родить ребенка. Березовская Е.П. — 290 стр. International Academy of Healthy Life. Торонто, Канада, 2024. (Ebook ISBN: 978-0-9867786-7-4)
25. Angel. Olena Berezovska. — 256 p. International Academy of Healthy Life. Toronto, Canada, 2024. (Ebook ISBN: 978-0-9867786-8-1)
26. Ангел. Березовська О.П. — 270 стор. International Academy of Healthy Life. Торонто, Канада, 2024. (Print ISBN 978-0-9867786-9-8, Ebook ISBN 978-1-997797-00-5)
27. Grandma Lena's Bedtime Stories. Olena Berezovska. — 154 p. International Academy of Healthy Life. Toronto, Canada, 2024. (Print ISBN: 978-1-0691603-0-0)
28. Привіт, малюк! Як пройти четвертий триместр без турбот і хвилювань. Березовська О.П. — 290 стор. International Academy of Healthy Life. Торонто, Канада, 2024. (Print ISBN: 978-1-0691603-3-1)
29. Growing Up Strong: A Guide to Girls' Health and Well-Being. Olena Berezovska. — 422 p. International Academy of Healthy Life. Toronto, Canada, 2025. (Print ISBN: 978-1-0691603-4-8, Ebook: 978-1-0694544-6-1)
30. Вечірні казочки бабусі Олени. Березовська О.П. — 180 стор. International Academy of Healthy Life. Toronto, Canada, 2025 (Print ISBN: 978-1-0691603-1-7)
31. Вечерние сказки бабушки Лены. Березовская Е.П. — 172 стр. International Academy of Healthy Life. Toronto, Canada, 2025 (Ebook ISBN: 978-1-0691603-2-4).

32. The Curious Escapades of a Corpse Named Jack. Book 1. Olena Berezovska. — 190 p. International Academy of Healthy Life. Toronto, Canada, 2025 (Print ISBN: 978-1-0691603-5-5, Ebook IBSN: 978-1-997797-02-9)
33. Основи здоров'я дівчаток: Практичний путівник для батьків. Березовська О. — 570 стор. International Academy of Healthy Life. Toronto, Canada, 2025 (Print ISBN: 978-1-0691603-6-2, Ebook: 978-1-0694544-7-8)
34. The Curious Escapades of a Corpse Named Jack. Book 2. Olena Berezovska. — 112 p. International Academy of Healthy Life. Toronto, Canada, 2025 (Print ISBN: 978-1-0691603-7-9, Ebook ISBN: 978-1-997797-03-6)
35. Hormonal Intelligence: How Hormones Shape Health and Well-being. Olena Berezovska. — 478 p. International Academy of Healthy Life. Toronto, Canada, 2025 (Print ISBN: 978-1-0691603-8-6, Ebook IBSN: 978-1-0694544-4-7)
36. Все про гормони: Таємна мова вашого тіла. Олена Березовська. — 460 с. International Academy of Healthy Life. Торонто, Канада, 2025 (Print ISBN: 978-1-0691603-9-3, Ebook IBSN: 978-1-0694544-5-4)
37. Дивовижні пригоди трупа на ім'я Джек: Книга 1. Олена Березовська. — 180 с. International Academy of Healthy Life. Торонто, Канада, 2025 (Print ISBN: 978-1-0694544-0-9, Ebook IBSN: 978-1-997797-04-3)
38. Підготовка до вагітності: Посібник з усвідомленого батьківства. Олена Березовська. — 468 с. International Academy of Healthy Life. Торонто, Канада, 25 травня 2025 (Print ISBN: 978-1-0694544-41-6, Ebook IBSN: 978-1-0694544-8-5)
39. DIY Bestseller: How to Write, Publish, and Market Your Book in the AI Era. Olena Berezovska. — 432 p. International Academy of Healthy Life. Toronto, Canada, 2025. (Print ISBN: 978-1-0694544-2-3, Ebook IBSN: 978-1-997797-01-2)

40. Mind Over Muscle: A Journal for Teen Athletes. Olena Berezovska. — 56 p. International Academy of Healthy Life. Toronto, Canada, 2025. (Print ISBN: 978-1-0694544-3-0, Ebook IBSN: 978-1-0694544-3-0)
41. Kopf schlägt Muskeln: Ein Journal für jugendliche Athleten. Olena Berezovska. — 58 p. International Academy of Healthy Life. Toronto, Canada, 2025. (Print ISBN: 978-1-997797-07-4 , Ebook ISBN: 979-8-231304-94-3)
42. After Delivery: A Doctor's Guide to Postpartum Healing and Recovery. Olena Berezovska. – 400 p. International Academy of Healthy Life. Toronto, Canada, 2025 (Print ISBN: 978-1-997797-08-1, Ebook ISBN: 978-1-997797-09-8).

www.ingramcontent.com/pod-product-compliance
Lightning Source LLC
LaVergne TN
LVHW090307210926
848480LV00001B/165

9798232951443